# MENTALK
## HEALTH

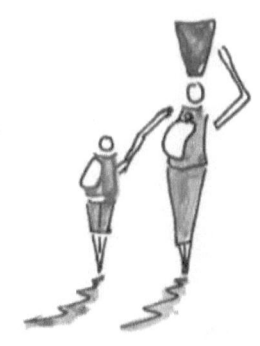

EMMANUEL OWUSU

authorHOUSE®

AuthorHouse™ UK
1663 Liberty Drive
Bloomington, IN 47403 USA
www.authorhouse.co.uk
Phone: 0800.197.4150

Published by AuthorHouse  04/05/2018

ISBN: 978-1-5462-9058-2 (sc)
ISBN: 978-1-5462-9086-5 (hc)
ISBN: 978-1-5462-9059-9 (e)

# CONTENTS

# PREFACE

*Mentalk Health* is a book full of stories.

Remarkably brave and inspiring stories from men from all walks of life who speak candidly about mental health issues.

Mentalk health is the fourth book in the series about the theme, Mental Health. It is preceded by *'My Psychosis Story'*, *'Let's Talk Mental Health'* and *'The Arts and Mental Health.'* Within the book, amongst many, Doctors, Footballer, Business systems and Production Manager, a Territorial Army Reserve, Psychiatric Epidemiologist, Personal Trainer, a Sustainability Consultant and a National Professional Advisor in Forensic Mental Health to name a few reveals their stories of post-traumatic stress disorder, depression, anxiety, severe stress, bipolar disorder and Psychosis. The book comprises of transcripts of recordings from interviews I conducted with various people on the subject matter.

Speaking to these amazing individuals aided me in my own recovery process. Having been diagnosed with psychosis, a severe mental health disorder a few years ago, I am still going through the emotions of dealing with this illness. Listening to their stories coping mechanisms that I now use to improve my health.

"Men have a problem with opening up
and speaking about their health"

The inspiration for this book was a result of learning that suicidal rates amongst men are '**3 times higher in the UK**' than women. This led me to investigate why this is and ask what, if anything, can be done about it?

A study conducted by the University of Misouri where more than 2000 school aged children participated revealed that boys and girls are fundamentally different when it comes to talking about their feelings. While girls love nothing more than to yap at length about what's bothering them, boys tend to keep quiet -- and not because they're embarrassed; they **just see it as a waste of time.**

Dr. Amanda Rose who lead the research suggested that this perception often carries onto manhood. She stated that "men may be more likely to think about talking about their problems which will make the problem feel bigger and they believe that engaging in different activities will take their minds off the problem"

This is a very worrying discovery. During my recovery process from Psychosis, I was prescribed a course of Cognitive behavioural therapy (CBT). According to the NHS, '*Cognitive behavioural therapy (CBT) is a talking therapy that can help you manage your problems by changing the way you think and behave. It's most commonly used to treat anxiety and depression, but can be useful for other mental and physical health problems.*

Having experienced first-hand the benefits of talking therapy, I am a big advocate of talking through problems. This involves the process of opening up and sharing issues with others instead of harbouring it internally which can result in the problem getting to unmanageable levels.

In an age where there is still much stigma associated with mental illness, this is a deeply powerful book which is written in the hope that it raises mental health and associated wider health issues. Importantly, it encourages men to talk about our mental health which can help to eradicate the stigma and prevent the alarming high rates of men dying as a result of mental health issues and associated wider health issues.

It is my hope that by reading this book, you are inspired by the brave stories. If you are experiencing some form of mental health issue or know someone who is, please understand that by being bold and talking about it with someone who understand, can help.

Throughout the book, I make references to sources of information regarding different mental health illnesses. These can be found on <u>www.nhs.uk</u>.

*How can we change the stigma?*


*"Time"*


*"Education"*


**Stories**

# SUICIDE IN THE UK AND ROI

*"In order to understand and prevent suicide, it is very important that suicide data is as accurate and as comprehensive as possible. Samaritans' Suicide Statistics Report 2017 provides details of the national suicide rates for the United Kingdom (UK) and Republic of Ireland (ROI). There is also additional information about how to understand and interpret suicide statistics, because it's not always as straight forward as looking at the actual numbers."*

*"Suicide is complex. It usually occurs gradually, progressing from suicidal thoughts, to planning, to attempting suicide and finally dying by suicide."*

**Source:** International Association for Suicide Prevention

## Key trends from the Samaritans Suicide Statistics Report 2017

6,188 suicides were registered in the UK and 451 in the Republic of Ireland.

**The highest suicide rate in the UK was for men aged 40–44.**

The highest suicide rate in the Republic of Ireland was for men aged 25–34 (with an almost identical rate for men aged 45–54).

Rates have increased in the UK (by 3.8%), England (by 2%), Wales (61.8%) and Northern Ireland (18.5%) since 2014 – however increases in Wales and Northern Ireland may be explained by inconsistencies in the processes for recording suicides in these countries.

Male rates remain consistently higher than female suicide rates across the UK and Republic of Ireland – most notably 5 times higher in Republic of Ireland and around 3 times in the UK.

## UK Suicide rates

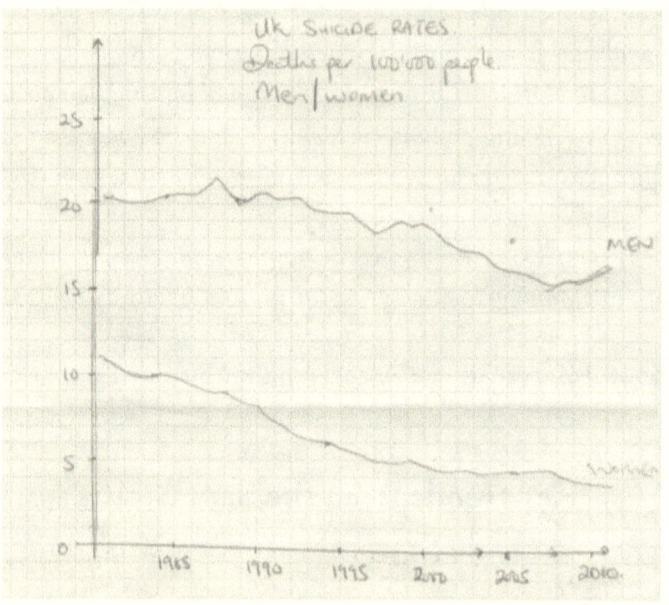

**Source:** *Office of National Statistics*

https://www.theguardian.com/society/2015/oct/31/social-media-campaign-male-suicide

Women have higher rates of depression, post-traumatic stress disorder (PTSD) and stress related problems than men however no one has yet to pinpoint this to a biological reason for the difference.

# Suicidal Thoughts

Suicide is the act of intentionally ending your life.

If you're reading this because you have, or have had, thoughts about taking your life, it's important you ask someone for help. It's probably difficult for you to see at this time, but you're not alone and not beyond help.

Many people who've had suicidal thoughts say they were so overwhelmed by negative feelings they felt they had no other option. However, with support and treatment they were able to allow the negative feelings to pass.

## If you're worried someone is suicidal

If you're worried that someone you know may be considering suicide, try to encourage them to talk about how they are feeling. Listening is the best way to help. Try to avoid offering solutions and try not to judge. If they've previously been diagnosed with a mental health condition, such as depression, you can speak to a member of their care team for help and advice.

## Why some people take their life

There's no single reason why someone may try to take their life, but certain things can increase the risk.

A person may be more likely to have suicidal thoughts if they have a mental health condition, such as depression, bipolar disorder or schizophrenia. Misusing alcohol or drugs and having poor job security can also make a person more vulnerable.

It's not always possible to prevent suicidal thoughts, but keeping your mind healthy with regular exercise, healthy eating and maintaining friendships can help you cope better with stressful or upsetting situations.

# THE VITRUVIAN MAN

By Leonardo da Vinci

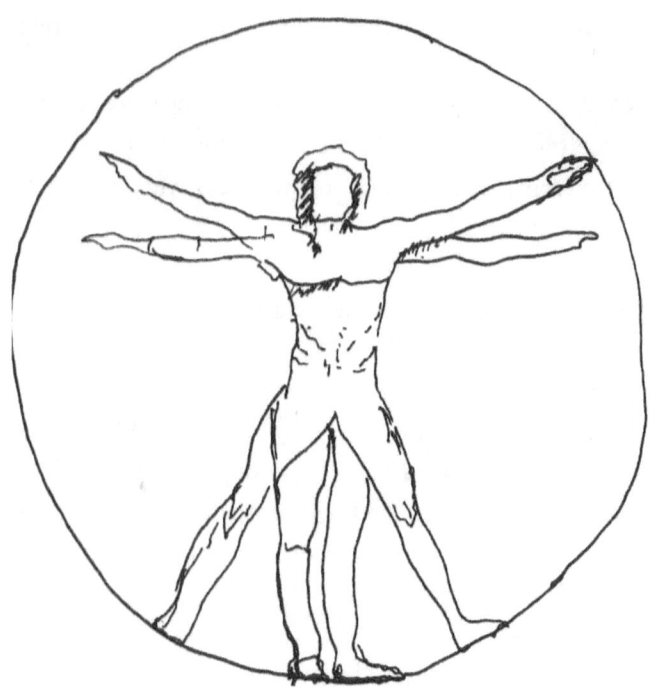

The Vitruvian man was created by Leonardo da Vinci in the late 15th century. Produced in pen and ink on paper, the drawing depicts two superimposed positions of a male figure with his arms and legs apart and simultaneously inscribed in a circle and square. The drawing is sometimes known as *the Canon of Proportions* or, *Proportions of Man*. Da Vinci had a keen interest in proportion. This drawing represents a keystone of Leonardo's attempts to draw comparisons between man and nature. The proportional relationship of the parts of the man reflects universal creation. Da Vinci's concept of the Vitruvian Man, represented in the drawing is one of the most popular world icons.

He spent much of his life searching for connections between patterns in nature and the structure of the human body. He was obsessed by the idea of making the universal measurement of the body and soul. In his notes which accompany the drawing, he proclaimed that *"Man is the model of the world."*

I'm fascinated by this drawing on many fronts, because Leonardo da Vinci is a creative genius who I hold in high regard. I often try to reproduce many of his anatomical studies of the human body as a pass time. As a man of many talents, he had interesting concepts and philosophies about the *'mechanics of man.'*

For me, this drawing is relevant to the subject of the book, not simply because the matter is man but because of the notion of man being this perfect *'model of the world'*

What pressure does this place upon our shoulders as men? The idea that the proportions of nature can in some way be better understood by studying the proportions of man is remarkable.

When I look at body parts such as my biceps, fingers, feet, thighs, shoulders and neck, can I truly have a better understanding of the works of nature and the universe?

This is incredibly challenging for me to fathom.

This idea of man possessing perfect anatomical figure to which we can relate to nature brings up the question whether this seeps beyond just a physical relationship. Can we relate whether there is a connection with a man's soul and emotions and nature itself.

Is there a harmony?

If there is an accord then this reveals a notion of the power of man. When I study this sketch, I see a fantastic attempt that not only asks a mathematical question about proportions, but asks more intrinsic questions about the power of man beyond the physical structure. The simple message I take from this sketch is that us men are powerful! So powerful that if we understand our physical, emotional and spiritual make up, we can possess an understanding of the mechanics of nature.

What a mind-blowing notion.

# DEPRESSION

**Depression is more than simply feeling unhappy or fed up for a few days.**

Most people go through periods of feeling down, but when you're depressed you feel persistently sad for weeks or months, rather than just a few days.

Some people think that depression is trivial and not a genuine health condition. They're wrong – it is a real illness with real symptoms. Depression isn't a sign of weakness or something you can "snap out of" by "pulling yourself together".

According to the NHS, depression is a low mood that lasts for a long time (2 weeks), and affects your everyday life. (NHS Choices, 2016). According to the International Classification of Diseases (ICD-10), diagnostic criteria for depression uses an agreed list of 10 depressive symptoms. These include:

## Key symptoms

- persistent sadness or low mood; and/or
- loss of interests or pleasure
- fatigue or low energy

at least one of these, most days, most of the time for at least 2 weeks. If any of above symptoms are present, please ask about **associated symptoms:**

- disturbed sleep
- poor concentration or indecisiveness
- low self-confidence

- poor or increased appetite
- suicidal thoughts or acts
- agitation or slowing of movements
- guilt or self-blame

The 10 symptoms then define the degree of depression and management is based on the particular degree.

- **not depressed** (fewer than four symptoms)
- **mild depression** (four symptoms)
- **moderate depression** (five to six symptoms)
- **severe depression** (seven or more symptoms, with or without psychotic symptoms) symptoms should be present for a month or more and every symptom should be present for most of every day.

In its mildest form, depression can mean just being in low spirits. It doesn't stop you leading your normal life but makes everything harder to do and seem less worthwhile. At its most severe, depression can be life-threatening because it can make you feel suicidal or simply give up the will to live. (Mind, 2000).

The good news is that with the right treatment and support, most people with depression can make a full recovery.

## How to tell if you have depression

Depression affects people in different ways and can cause a wide variety of symptoms.

They range from lasting feelings of unhappiness and hopelessness, to losing interest in the things you used to enjoy and feeling very tearful. Many people with depression also have symptoms of anxiety.

There can be physical symptoms too, such as feeling constantly tired, sleeping badly, having no appetite or sex drive, and various aches and pains.

The symptoms of depression range from mild to severe. At its mildest, you may simply feel persistently low in spirit, while severe depression can make you feel suicidal, that life is no longer worth living.

Most people experience feelings of stress, unhappiness or anxiety during difficult times. A low mood may improve after a short period of time, rather than being a sign of depression.

# CHAT OVER A CAN OF COKE

I suffer from anxiety and deep depression. I have periods where my mood just snaps which means I can go from 0 – 100 in seconds. I have self-harmed quite a few times and I can get angry very easily. As a person, I am very much hard work. Relationships are pretty much a no go area for me because people can't handle me because I can be that much of a problem.

**Have you tried to seek help?**

I've had Cognitive Behavioural Therapy (CBT) which was effective whilst I was having it. It was amazing doing the programme. But whilst I'm good at the theoretical aspect and practice whilst I'm on the programme, afterward, I tail of. I lose focus and it seems like everything I learn loses value. I start to feel like I can't do it anymore and I forget what I've learnt.

**What techniques did CBT introduce you to?**

I learnt techniques which include 'Compartmentalising' 'Rationalising', 'Black and White', 'Putting it in a box'. It introduced me to simple techniques about how to deal with my issues such as alternative ways to handle situations.

**What are the positives and negatives to CBT?**

The good thing is it gave me something to focus on and it gave me techniques that I hadn't thought of. I'd been so stuck in a rut of being overwhelmed. The bad point is, because of the mental health system we have in place right now, we don't really get follow ups. Therefore, after you've done the course, you're simply expected to implement it and just cope. In reality, it's not that easy because I know I'd like to be able to do things but I need something to stay with after I complete the course. This would give me some sort of back up.

## Notion of Hope and recovery

For some people, there is hope and it can be an effective solution to cope but it depends on your life. I say this because, if you live alone, there is no support system in place. Your GP is often busy and so sometimes you don't get referment and they don't chase it up. At the same time, you're so overwhelmed and depressed that you can't follow it up either. Yet they are telling you that you must refer yourself.

It can be hard to find the confidence to make the phone call to get that much needed additional help. That is a hard thing to do. If you don't have the support system, the confidence and the ability to look after and do something for yourself, then you're pretty much screwed. You can't do it so there's no hope there. A lot of people are stuck and fall through the cracks. I have fallen through the cracks in the mental health system.

People say they will get you support, send you this letter, put you on this course, so on and so forth. I'm a laid back guy so I don't really chase things up. I don't have the confidence in myself to do things. Months go by and then it's forgotten. You speak with one person and they don't actually communicate with the other person. Things don't go through the right channels. For instance, the Psychiatrist might not go through to the consultant and the consultants might not put it down to the doctor who speaks with the secretary to organise the appointment so you can get lost in the system. I have been lost in that system many times. I'm still lost in that system. I've been trying to get a lot of help for many things and it's taking months.

## What was your first experience like when you got help and what was that process like?

My doctor referred me for CBT. Fortunately for me, I got one near my local surgery. But I had one session and my therapist had a personal emergency so she had to stop the CBT. It meant I was left without any support for months as I had to wait again for somebody else to become available. Luckily, I did eventually get help again and resumed my therapy.

For me, like many people, there is a problem with the connection. We have to be able to connect with someone to be able to open up. Luckily, I got on really well with my CBT therapist. This allowed me to be open and honest with her. Otherwise if you cannot connect with someone, you won't be able to open up and get help.

Mental health is like this, you can tell who is ready to learn something and who is not. You'll either be in a really good place or a bad one.

## Stigma.

Now see, this is a very contentious place for me because I hate the stigma! This is one of the worst things in existence. It's not right. It's a wrong thing that exists. If you've got a broken arm, people notice it and you get sympathy which can mean support and help. If you're depressed, they say, "get on with it, what's the matter with you." You can't see a mental illness and people don't understand that. Even if you've got cancer, they see the physical effects when you're going through therapy such as the loss of hair. People get that. But if you're mentally unwell, people can't see the symptoms of that unless you're self-harming. You can become very good at hiding things so that can become hard to recognise. People don't notice people with mental health problems. People don't know what mental health problem is and they don't care.

The amount of children now with mental health problems is unimaginable. There isn't much help for them.

To be labelled with things like "you're a nutter", "you're a mad case" "look at you, you're a sicko", all because you have bipolar or multiple personality disorder. People take the piss out of that because they can't handle that.

**There is a massive stigma toward it, it's disgusting and it must stop because it's evil!**

**What are some of the most useful ways we can address the stigma and move on?**

We must learn to be open and straightforward with people. We must stand up and keep fighting the stigma! We must be able to say, I've got a mental illness, so what? We've just got to deal with it. It's got to be addressed legally. For instance in a job interview, people should not be able to discriminate against you. Mental illness must align with anti-decimation stances such as gender, race, religion and sexuality. We've all got to be on a level playing field. Mental health must be on that field as well. Just because you've got a mental health problem doesn't mean you can't perform your job.

You can still become a doctor or a surgeon if you have a mental health issue. You can do anything if you have a mental health difficulty. As long as you are on the right treatment, you can do anything! Just because someone might have bipolar doesn't stop them from doing their job.

For instance, I may have type 1 diabetes which means I have to take insulin. If I take my medication and I look after myself, that won't stop me from performing brain surgery. So having mental health condition shouldn't be a problem for anyone. People should treat it as normal.

"There is a massive stigma toward it, it's disgusting and it must stop because it's evil!"

"Just because you've got a mental health problem doesn't mean you can't perform your job."

*"To be labelled with things like "you're a nutter", "you're a mad case" "look at you, you're a sicko", all because you have bipolar or multiple personality disorder. People take the piss out of that because they can't handle that."*

"We must stand up and
keep fighting the stigma!"

# CONVERSATION WITH L.O

**What's your personal experience with mental
health issues, if you have had any?**

I have, according to the NHS you probably just call it a classic case of
standard depression.

**You used the word standard there...**

I know there's no such thing as standard, but quite a lot of my recovery
was without doctor inference but they were aware. If I looked at myself
deep down, I could probably say it started or I was aware of it when I was
fourteen or fifteen. I only really had the tools to deal with my depression
when I was twenty-two. To this day, I'm better than ever but I would still
say that cloud still kind of exists. I thought it would be wrong to say that
I'm cured, I have it under control is probably a better way to describe
what I am right now.

**What do you think was the cause?**

I was aware of these feelings for a long time. I didn't really know what
it was until I was about eighteen and I went to university. My initial
coping mechanism was always to ignore myself and focus on others. Up
to the age of eighteen, there was always someone or something I was
always pouring my attention into, "don't feel so bad, here let me help
you through your problems". When I went to University, I left London.
I realised I didn't have anyone else's problems to solve. There wouldn't
be any real trigger moment. It was not a case of "Oh one day I fell off
a tree and hit my head", or "my girlfriend broke my heart". It was to do
with a lot of little things of me putting myself second. Ensuring that
others needs are cared for before ensuring my own one. Also, perhaps

low self-confidence played a role. I was a chubby kid, and I still think I am a little bit of a chubby guy now in my opinion.

My partner says I have a little bit of body dysmorphia. If I think of the right size I'm 6'3' I weigh 110kgs (17/18 stone), little bit of fat there but there's quite a lot of muscle. I'm a strong person but I see myself as a very average sized human being on the outside if I look at myself in mirrors.

A very good friend and I were on the bus one day. We always used to fight on the bus as we all used to do as kids, and one time he said, "Oh you're so big for no reason". That cut me. Because of that, the next day I went to the gym and found out what a barbell looked like and started that kind of journey.

I do digress, but it was one of those things. In the early years I was focusing on other people when I wasn't feeling great, when I was not feeling happy. Maybe I'm thinking if there was a pure trigger, when I was fourteen my parents divorced. I remember my mother giving me St John's Wort, which is a type of herbal medicine, which is said to be able to help with depression. However, I didn't know what I was taking. So, I get to eighteen and go to University out of London. None of my friends went there. There weren't many other people like me at University and you end up sitting in a room by yourself.

## What do you mean when you say people like you? Beliefs, stature?

All of it. The university I went to, what I believe, had the most amount of private school kids in the country. There was a very low black demographic, and you put the two together and you stick out like a sore thumb automatically. There weren't many black people, or people that had a similar upbringing to so it was very hard to find people like me.

I studied Electrical Engineering and I was the only black individual on my course out of a cohort of about 200 to 250. There was a high percentage of Indians and Chinese people, and there were some Nigerians that I'd come across, but the only thing we really shared in common was our skin colour. There were a few British people on that course as well, we're talking 10 to 15 out of that cohort. Then you would have the odd spot of Europeans but it was really just Arabs, Indians and Chinese guys so there wasn't really a circle there. I guess my friends in my 1st year, there wasn't really many. I started playing sport at uni.

**Which sport?**

American football.

I started playing American Football. I remember the first session I think I was sick. In hindsight, I don't know if I was sick or just anxious but I missed that one. I came to the second session wondering if it was too late. I trotted up and the people I met there are some of my closest friends to this day. I don't know what I would have done without that sport even though it was a major cause of my sadness as well.

**You mentioned the causes, low self-esteem etc., but what were the symptoms in terms of moods and feeling?**

Some people call it "the blues", some people call it low mood, sadness. An insular feeling. When your friends say do you want to go out, you say not really. You wake up some days and it was a victory to just get out of bed because you just felt as if there were walls closing on top of you. You know of course there's no walls and I wouldn't know what claustrophobia feels like because I'm not claustrophobic but it would feel very stuffy inside, or a black cloud hanging upon you which represented itself in low confidence attributes. Not speaking loud enough, being excessively anxious, eve physically turning your body inwards to have that stereotypical low confidence posture. That makes you want to stay inside because at least when you stay inside you don't need to have any anxious thoughts about what other people think about you.

**Jumping a few steps forward. You are in a better place now. What was that process like in terms of getting you to where you are now? What did you do? What did people do?**

Do you know what didn't work for me? Medication.

**What medication did you have?**

Anti- depressants. I want to say they had me on Citalopram at first and then they moved me onto Fluoxetine (Prozac).

**How long were you on these for?**

So, if you go back and I think my time in years. I ended up doing a 5-year course at Uni, not because I wanted to, but because I had to interrupt. 1 year for depression and 1 year for Ta sports injury. If I think back properly, it was my 3rd year that I was fully medicated.

**Did you go and get help yourself or did someone suggest you do?**

I went on my own accord, so I had been going on my own accord for quite a while.

**To a hospital or to a councillor?**

A General PR actioner (GP). In my 1st year at Uni, I knew that something was wrong, but I didn't do anything about it. I remember missing 3 weeks of lectures and just told people that I was sick. My grades didn't suffer. My 2nd year grades did suffer. I went down from averaging 80s in the first year to being in the 50s. I've been unlucky that I have had very bad living situations in my Uni life. My 1st year there was a neighbour that had an affinity for too many drugs and threatened my life a couple of times. The 2nd year I lived with someone who was very dirty and didn't keep a clean space, so that kind of affected me because I didn't want to spend my time cleaning up his mess so I ended up avoiding the communal areas when possible. At the end of 2nd year I went to see a GP to get it sorted out, they mentioned medication.

The conversation was: I can go to counselling which had an 8 week waiting list on the NHS or I can use medication. And then I also got referred to my university's counsellor. One thing I want to put in now is that **you need to continue trying until you find something that works for you.** That's why I started medication, because I went to my first counselling session and she suggested medication alongside sessions with her. "Give it a go, we'll see what happens". At the end of the day and I was particularly iffy about it but I said why not.

The one thing I always think about depression is that it isn't being sad, **depression is feeling nothing almost.** The opposite of happiness isn't sadness, the opposite of happiness is apathy. All the medication did for me was make me feel more apathetic. It allowed me to get up yes, but things that I would enjoy before the meds I wouldn't anymore. The little joy that I had was taken away from me by taking that medication.

I did a course of citalopram, didn't like it went to the GP again and got a new course.

## How long was that?

This was about a 6-8 week period. So, this is my second year of Uni, this is the 2nd half of it, nearer the exams that I had a course of Citalopram. Then I stopped taking them because I wanted to do my exams. I did my exams. Then I came back the next year and it was all the same so that's when I used Prozac instead that year but I was still the same. And the worst part was, my GP who I was working with the first time had left because she was having a baby.

I tried to find a GP but could never find someone but I landed a good counsellor that year. She was quite decent and honestly, we just spoke. Talked it through and I sat down for hours and wrote things down with that GP that's when CBT became a thing and that was probably the biggest help for myself.

We did quite a few workshops with similar people suffering at the University. Some were solo sessions. She also ran group sessions and invited me to go. We did some mindfulness sessions, we did some group CBT, we also did some solo talk therapy. A combination of all of those gave me quite a lot of tools and made me feel that I could do something.

The mistake I then made was going back on the medication again because it was getting to the exams and I wanted to make sure that I could pass. I was not really enjoying engineering that much, I like it but I questioned whether I really loved it and could make a career out of it.

I couldn't see myself working in engineering when I finished is probably the best way to put it but I enjoyed the studies. I thought okay let's go back on the medication to see if that will help. I particularly remember it because I had a panic attack in one of the exam. I don't remember exactly why but I think I thought I was in exam A but I was sitting exam B and I literally broke down inside the hall. I left the exam hall and had a 15-minute breathing fit before coming back into the room.

This is my winter exams in my 3rd year and the invigilator was encouraging me to return and finish my exams and just do the best you can. After that experience, I realized that I could either sit down and finish the course or I can go and actually fix myself and so **I decided to go and fix myself.** For me, this represented me sitting down in the middle of a bed crying my heart out and not actually achieving anything until my mother basically gave me some tough love and now I'm very thankful for her for doing that.

**So fixing yourself was taking time out
from Uni? The whole year?**

Half a year. Going back to London, back to the house. I couldn't take a whole year off and come back because the way my course is written. In that year I lost some access to talking to the counsellor however, before I left she gave me some tools and programs so that I could continue my CBT. After feeling sorry for myself for a bit, I then started doing work.

I was a security guard for that summer, just working, long hours. Getting myself outside was probably the biggest thing because sitting indoors wouldn't help anything. So I remember working 29 days out of 3, 12 hour shifts, and I still felt good because I was doing something. I was tired, but I was doing something and I had a focus in mind as well.

**With regards to CBT, what are some of
the pros and cons in your opinion?**

I don't think there are that many cons about it to be honest. If you look at mental health you have got two different types of issues. That's not the right word but it's the word I'm going to use. You have issues where **you die about overthinking** and then there are issues where **you die through over imagination.**

**Clarification…Imagination, thinking?**

So, the difference between somebody who is bi-polar is that one day they are depressed and they over think. They think themselves through negative thought process and there are other days where they are manic… or if someone is uneducated they look ultra-impulsive; or they are not actually thinking but just exploding outwards. I'm not sure If I can verbalise it correctly, but the way I see it, as in both are poor because one you dig yourself into an early grave and on the other side you have no inhibition what so ever. So maybe we should rephrase that and say inhibition and in-inhibition as opposed to thinking and imagination?

**Yes.**

So you start thinking and you think and you think and you are almost too aware and there are other times where you lose all your inhibitions and go crazy. And CBT tends to not work for the latter, because you're not thinking and obviously for it to work you need to be actively aware.

You have your cycle of thoughts and the key is to catch at a certain point. For example, let's say my problems is that I have a lot of vices apart from hard drugs I did most of them. There was a time where the roulette table was my best friend, where alcohol was my best friend, there was a time where weed was my best friend, a time where Dominos pizza was my best friend. CBT would make me aware that 'Oh wait, I have smoked a bag but had no reason to. Why are you doing this? Ok, what are you feeling? Let's fix it.' Or I look around my room and say 'wait why have I got 10 boxes of Dominos and a couple of take away boxes out here. ok let's correct it.

Whereas without that CBT you would not be aware of these things and aware of what you do because you never really capture your initial thought. You don't catch it in the 'I feel crappy thought'. You usually catch it after you've done something which is your coping mechanism. You have your thought.

'I don't like myself,
Action = I'm going to drink so I feel better about myself
Result = This makes me feel crappy.

Let's make it a real analogy. A real negative thought process is:

*'I have an exam tomorrow and I haven't studied yet,
I feel crap about it so I'm going to try and study
but I can't focus on my studies because I'm really
not in a good mental health space
so that makes me feel bad about myself because I can't
study because I'm in a bade mental health state,*

So, I follow that loop a couple of times. I can't study any more so what am I going to do?

Well I'm stressed ------ (insert de-stressor of choice)------ Let's say your de-stressor of choice is to go and have a drink.

so your cycle goes from.

> *I need to study,*
> *I'm going to try and study*
> *but I can't study because I'm in a bad mental health state*
> *so I'm going to try harder to study.*
> *Going to try to study, can't study,*
> *bad mental health state*
> *I'm going to have a drink*
> *so I can see if I can get better*

so I can't do that I'm going to drink, drink makes me feel better, I have a drink, drink doesn't make me feel better but I don't know that because I feel better but in reality it doesn't make me feel better so let me have another drink, let me try and study, can't study, cool now I'm drunk. Wake up the next morning 'what am I doing here?' Let me go and try to study again. You can go through these patterns and that a very high level one because they usually are more serious and I am very good at noticing them. Now usually when I'm sat I just notice the feeling already.

### So you are able to capture it in the process?

Before I couldn't and only realised after the fact, for example I spent all my student loan in the casino, but now I can catch it at that initial feeling and fix it before I do anything negative.

### How do you capture this within the thought process?

Time.

It sucks, but time.

**The more and more I practice the more I'm aware of my thoughts,** the better I got at recognising when something was about to happen. All I do right now is say 'hi partner, not feeling so great today'. If I'm at work and I feel like that, no one at work knows, but I will just call it off mentally for the day. I won't go 100% for the day, I'll call it off, I'll leave on time. Go home probably watch a couple of episodes of Gilmore Girls and I'm good to go.

**Gilmore girls!!!**
**My man, I enjoy that show!!**

The new 4-episode series is on Netflix right now.

**Digression**

Right now, I've gotten to the stage where, not all the time, I mostly catch it at that initial negative thought. They are never actually caused by something happening.

I currently work in recruitment, which is a fun job because you get paid to matchmake for people but humans makes it more difficult than it should be and nobody appreciates what you do. You kind of get used to being 2nd class citizens and your aim is to ultimately make it as easy as possible, to try and change your perception of you so that you can operate better, so that they can operate better. But that's another conversation about how poor the recruitment industry is working right now.

You get used to having these negative outcomes and then you **recognise** the difference between negative outcome, 'I couldn't get that piece of business', or negative outcome, 'my candidate didn't get a job', or negative outcome, 'Oh I might be dropping' and you recognise the difference. I think it might have actually helped me in my recognition.

**You're using the R word. I suspect that's a therapy thing. The 3 R's? Recognition, Rationalise, Replace, does that ring a bell?**

I remember that from my CBT. I used recognise purely from my American football background. From play recognition. Before play happens, you see people in a certain situation and then after that first couple of steps you should be recognising what is going to happen so you know how to act.

Likewise, the whole emphasis of CBT is to recognise the feeling if you can or recognise the actions you are about to have.

Let's say for example you are a attractive lady and you don't see yourself as beautiful. Someone could say something mean about you and that sends you into a cycle, but your form of coping is to go to a club, get as drunk as possible and find a guy who is going to say pretty things about you and take you home.

You don't always realise that until you are back at home. The next morning you are looking at this ugly guy with a massive beard and you think to yourself 'what did I do here?' and then you get into your own negative patterns.

Now if you go back to that same scenario, you have two ways to think about it. You either fix your self- esteem issues or you can recognise when you are about to have that drink before you go outside because you don't want to get into that situation. Sometimes it's harmless depending what your vice is, what your mechanism is. But your mechanism can make you feel worse in the long term and you want to be able to catch it as soon as possible. You always want to catch it as soon as possible, you want to see it.

Because what if your coping mechanism is drugs and you can't catch it? You just go down the rabbit hole from softer to harder drugs until you can find the answer by the time you've realised, you are addicted to a drug, and now your work is not actually to fix yourself, but your addiction at the end of the day.

In a nutshell **with CBT you have to be incredibly self-aware** which is very hard for someone who is going through, at least my version of depression. Because quite a lot of the time you have your own internal dialogue with yourself which isn't always pretty dialogue, and for you to go and beat yourself up mentally in your head. On the other hand, recognising that you are doing that is not easy.

It's not your nature.

# Caveman instincts

Almost as such. Funny how we are in a society where everybody is supposed to be equal but then your stereotypes positive male traits such as being strong, brave, adventurous, outgoing always tends to come up, right?

As in depression is not a thing full stop. In this sense of how I feel the public tend to see it. Of course, I know it's real and many people do, but you always get examples where you should 'man up' is what you always hear a lot, or yes you'll be better just go and watch some TV or have some ice cream, I don't feel like that.

A great example is your life is good why do you feel like that? Or what do you have to be depressed about? Now you can compound the fact that, at least socially, you're allowed to be more emotional as a woman. It's more acceptable to cry as a woman compared to a man.

I don't cry, I just can't do it. I think maybe I've cried twice in the past 10 years. Apparently, I'm not a pretty crier, but that's another story for another day.

I would say **it sucks to be depressed as a man** but **it sucks to be depressed full stop.** The difference is I guess because women are allowed to explore their feelings more often. If seems more acceptable for them to get the help more often.

I don't know, because it's funny you mentioned that group course. With CBT there were 12 people, there were 3 guys and both of the other guys were not 'macho' men. You put me there and at that time I was the fittest in my life, muscles all over, sitting down saying I feel depressed. The image just doesn't work right. When you think depressed you think of a little frail person. I'm not sure if you agree or disagree with that sentence...

**Yes I'm with you.**

Whether they are male or female is a different question. It's one of those things where, and I think it's probably why there is a much higher suicide rate with men than with women. It's probably because by the time quite a lot of men actually realise they should have got this help, it's too late and we're talking about the CBT cycles earlier, the cycles and cycles and cycles, every cycle is an opportunity to make a change and because there is so little where you just get to a situation where you feel there is no escape.

Not to mention with our gender stereotypes it's okay if a woman doesn't necessarily feel like doing a 40 hour week if they want to go and look after the kids. For a man however, not really. What's this paternity leave you talk about? You see people go on maternity leave for 6-8 months, Men at my work place go on paternity leave for 2 weeks max and they're still on their phones while on paternity leave.

These are all things that won't change for the next 20 years. It's one of those things you can't just go and say or decree and it automatically gets better. The short of it is that **men need to talk more and be honest.** I've found the biggest changes in my life apart from the awareness and the power of CBT is being as honest as I can be within reason.

Not brutally honest, a good book AJ Jacobs I wrote a book called 'My Life as an Experiment' and he dedicates a chapter to radical honesty. It's a concept where you say what's on your mind whenever which doesn't always go down so well. By being honest, loving myself and not caring what other people think.

**Afro Caribbean men…**

Ah ha, lets compound it. When I mentioned your frail person, was it a frail white guy? It wasn't a frail African or a frail Caribbean. Those strength psyches just worsen almost. As in if you are a guy you are supposed to be strong. **If you are African you are definitely supposed to be the strong guy.** It's neigh on impossible to be a soft black guy because, depending on the circles you roll in, you are automatically given the gay stigma term. Or you are victimized by other people in your circle. The sad part about it is that I don't think there is much you can change because stereotypes are stereotypes.

Some of them are true, some of them aren't. It would be great if tomorrow you could sit down and have 50 black people talk about depression. I mean to myself, with the exception of youself, my partner, my parents and a couple of very close friends, not many people know. It's almost in my head, what do they gain to know? I would rather they have an image of a strong black guy than a guy with feelings who can't always get up in the morning because he feels crappy about himself for no apparent reason.

**Change. Stigma. Stereotypes.**


**How do we break down the walls?**

Time,
Education,
Stories

# Time.

Everybody always says that if we all get together and put our minds together it will change our minds or something. No, it can't. The perfect example is smoking.

We all know smoking is bad for your health. Some people find the smoke kind of pleasant, and some of them don't, yet they still smoke. What's changed? It hasn't really been the fact that cigarettes are costing more money and they put ugly packaging on it. It's that you've put the theory that cigarettes are bad and they are harmful and push that through governmental policy backed by scientific study and then you educate the children to know that cigarettes are bad. This will ensure that when your 5 year old says 'Daddy I don't like it when you smoke', 'Mummy smoking is going to kill you and I want to see you when I grow old' you have that chain of guilt. Now those older people, those who are 20,30,40 are now 40,50, 60 in 20 years' time and maybe they have stopped smoking now because they've got heart problems, or they can't run as fast because smoking have got them.

Some of them of course are still smoking and still smoke 20 a day until the old age of 97, but now you are talking about your current 20 year olds, who have kids who were indoctrinated in this 'smoking is bad' are now 20 and they are not smoking. Now on TV you don't nearly see as much smoking because that's not what you do anymore. So, it's the time thing. You look at America with the whole black lives matters stuff, it's been 50 years since Martin Luther King? At least 150 years since the end of slavery.

You look at that country they still haven't gotten over it yet. They're still trying to educate the people.

**It will take time for that to happen.**

# Education.

If you aren't putting it out there, how do you think people will change. Why would people think mental health is actually a thing if you're not letting people know that mental health is actually a thing.

If somebody has not gone through mental health issue they will not know the effects. At least with a physical ailment, if you see someone has really bad eczema you can see their skin peel. If you haven't been in that situation you can still empathize with them because you can see.

One thing I like to do is to watch people arm wrestle. Which is not great, but I watch it to remind myself never to do it. You will see these two guys and one will snap right in the middle of the forearm and everybody just winces and you can associate there. However, no one can really empathize with mental illness unless they've actually been there. Its why you have questions like **how do I help somebody who has a mental illness.** You don't have questions like how do I help someone that has broken a leg. Hopefully we get to a stage where we don't have that and **the way we educate people is through stories.**

# Stories.

Honestly, right now I wouldn't feel brave enough to tell my story. There are many people who do and that's the best way to explain it, how else do you make 15-16 year old black kids feel that it's okay to feel like that than when you put somebody who was in their shoes.

Again, you can talk about the whole being colour neutral but at the end of the day if I'm playing a video game and I get to make my character look like something, I'm going to make my character black because that's what I am. It's easier for somebody to gravitate to somebody who looks like them or has their upbringing.

It's usually in the poorer places in our country where it's more prevalent, most likely because the thought of it, life tends to be harder because they have more problems. Some could argue with me that everyone has problems, and I can understand that if your parent makes a combined total of £25k a year or your dad makes £250k, you're going to have problems. Although relatively, both problems will be on a similar level, on an absolute level, you will consider not being able to go on holiday much less of a problem than not having means to eat. Going through that hardship means that you need to have that mental capabilities ready so you can deal with that external stress.

# Faith.

It's hard to say because I can't just go and say yes and I can't actually say no because there is a statue of John Paul II in the corner in my house. Because I guess like myself, I am a natural introvert and my faith is very internal, and when I was at my lowest of lows I wasn't saying 'well God is going to get me out of this'.

Right now, do I thank God for everything that I have? Yes. It's one of those things that I'm aware of and sometimes it's helped me to have a different shift on focus, but I can't say the reason why I beat depression was because of my undying faith to God/Jesus, because deep down that wasn't the driver, I wasn't saying 'oh if I pray more I get better'.

It might just be because of my nature. I believe that God gives you the power and the tools to work wonders, I don't believe that God does things for you. Therefore when people say for example 'It's a miracle, bless God, God did this for you' I say 'oh you kind of take away the credit'. He has had a major part in it, but he has given me or that person the tools to do that, and this person has worked hard and through their faith managed to achieve, now you go and belittle that and say it wasn't all you.

From the way I see, faith is like a multiplier. If somebody believes in the cause great enough they can do wonders, now if they believe in that faith and they're backed by God or their deity of choice, then they are even stronger.

I think it's a bit of an unfair advantage that people of faith have than those without faith, if they truly believe. one thing I haven't mentioned is that oh it's the devil or it's a curse, because it's not. **We are all unique, we all have our trials and tribulations and it's our job to figure it out how to deal with them in the best way possible.** I mean I'd probably say I suffer, or suffered depression depending on how you want to look at it because I had poor mental health processes and coping mechanisms not because I slept one day and the devil breathed fire in my mouth.

Some people again try to trivialize the human and over focus the supernatural. It's always you need to go to church more, you need to pray more. Your faith helps you get out of the trials and situations, but your faith is no outer power that is making you do that. I guess I almost see, when I talk about software development, almost like God is the architect and you are the developer, he creates the constructs and guidelines which you use to operate and gives you the tools that you need to do what you need to do and it's your job to go and do it if that makes sense.

I always think of my mum with this friend who was a very devout Christian. She has a child, incredibly poor, living just above the bread line and it's Christmas time so the pastor is clapping and everyone is clapping in the church and its donation time and the pastor is saying donations will feed your prayers.

Your prayers will set you free. And in my head I'm thinking this pastor is just getting you to donate so he can buy a brand new car mate, he's got an Audi but he wants a BMW. Anyway, she gives him £20 and then he takes the money looks at the money and it's not enough money, you need to donate more it's Christmas time. She gave the last £20 she had, the last £20 she had to the man. She goes home, no gas, no electric…it cuts off.

God will provide… Puts on the emergency, God will provide. It's Christmas time, it's cold, she's in the old house you know. She's got a hot water bottle at the foot of her bed to keep her warm and she feels a burning sensation and thinks the devil is testing her, "the devil is testing me"… she wakes up the next morning with a burnt foot, can't work for 12 days. Grade 2 skin burns, had to go to hospital couldn't work for 2 weeks. She is there thinking "God will provide."

No, if you had kept your £20, God already provided it, put that on your gas and electric. Then you wouldn't have needed the hot water bottle because you could have put the heat on for the rest of the night.

Now you have a water bottle in your bed and you feel heat, what's the simplest thing…it's not a supernatural power coming in and testing you. Have a look, if you haven't got water leaking on you then you can go and make any praise you want.

Back to that decision, she couldn't work for two weeks and you can say God will provide but did God provide there? I say he did long time ago.

Hope.

**What is hope to you, what does it mean, if anything,
and how does that link with mental health?**

Hope.

It is the most important thing.

Without hope then you have no chance.

If you don't believe there's going to be an end then
you need to find a way to get that hope.

**Hope is the thought that one day you will wake
up and there won't be a cloud anymore**

At least that's how it is when it comes to depression. Or the most classic sense that it is going to be better the next day. You are going to wake up and what you wish intrinsically is going to occur and I believe **hope is a pure mental thing.** You read studies and they talk about people who are optimistic will live maybe 10 years longer than people who are pessimistic. You will see people with cancer, cancer that isn't meant to be cured, pull through because they had a positive outlook. Because instead of them thinking 'I've got cancer, oh woe is me' actually saying 'I've got cancer, I'm going to beat this cancer'. That's true hope.

Without you being mentally invested in that you aren't going to get the results you want. It's hard because with depression you aren't mentally thinking the way that you should be thinking so it's harder to then channel that inner hope that I hope one day I'm not depressed because usually the thought process, instead of saying 'I hope one day I'm not depressed' is 'I hope one day this is all over'.

# The Chimp inside of me

I have bought a couple of books. One called The Chimp Paradox by Dr Steve Peters which has changed my life. It's about recognising the chimp inside your head. In a nutshell, in your mind you have three different thought processes. You've got the human, which is the intellectual, the person that thinks things through. You have the chimp that feels and is very emotional and erratic, and then you have the computer which is automatically stored. For example, you wake up in the morning, you do your bed, you brush your teeth. That's computer force, that's stored. You just do it.

Now the difference between the chimp thought and the human thought is this. Let's say you are a woman and your husband says that dress doesn't look good on you, the human will say 'why doesn't it look too good, what's wrong with the dress?' 'Oh I just don't like the colour on you'. The chimp may say 'why is he hating on me for, does it make me look fat?' something along those lines and jump to a conclusion. The challenge however is the computer is always faster than the chimp, and the chimp is always faster than the human. That's why whenever people get into arguments you think oh I wish I never said that. It's because it's not you it's a chimpanzee, and all the chimpanzee cares about, just like how a dog, or even a real chimpanzee is shelter, safety, and nourishment.

It doesn't care about the existential crisis going on in Syria, all it cares about is that it feels safe, that it's not going to be attacked, it's got enough food to eat, and a roof over its head. That book has really helped me to understand my thoughts because almost like CBT, quite a lot of those negative thoughts are the chimps thoughts.

I've said something to somebody and I didn't get the acquired reaction, I made a joke and they didn't laugh, do they hate me? Those are all chimp thoughts, and then depending on what version, if you've got anxious chimp your chimp says "maybe they hate me... should I say something nice about them... oh what should I do to make it better....oh I've messed up now they're not going to like me any more… I've messed up, I'm such a failure."

If you have an aggressive chimp the conversation may go "that guy is a massive dickhead, I'm not going to talk to him anymore" Maybe they just didn't find it funny? The book kind of gives you techniques and makes you aware of the patterns so that when your chimp thinks you say cut it, I'm not going to listen to the chimp.

The perfect example is road rage. Come on, you don't know the person in the other car might be a world champion UFC fighter, or might be walking around with an AK47 at the back of his car, but you feel brave enough to go in there and shout at him or her. Why? It's pure chimp talking. I don't think someone has ever sat down and rationally gone and said 'Oh that guy just carved me up, what I should do in order to make sure that that guy understands that his actions were wrong. Perhaps, I should get out of my car, knock on his window and say 'there sir, you carved me up, I'm going to mess with you, I'm going to shout at you until you realise and say sorry'.

No, the human goes and says "forget about that, maybe he has a meeting he has to rush to. I'm happy that I am safe, I'm good to go." The chimp goes and thinks this guy is trying to hurt me, this guy is trying to harm my life.

That book has changed my life. It has helped me to slow down, understand and be calm and collected and seem almost too rational. That's probably also a reason why I've managed to be able to recognise that feeling a bit better because I can recognise when that chimp is talking inside of me. **My chimp is an anxious, depressed chimp.**

The second one is The Power of Habit by Charles Duhigg, and that book is about changing the way you do things and implementing the habits. These are things you talk about, things that help with depression, stuff like exercise is a big one, meeting with people, and that just helps with the habits.

Before we started I was talking about one of the stresses in life is making too many decisions and the key to keeping yourself as calm as possible and not getting that burnout is to make as little decisions as possible and to automate as much as what you do.

For me as a habit, I've just moved to a new house and I needed to start going back to the gym so when I wake up my clock goes off at the same time, I get up and do exactly the same thing. I go out to the gym every day for a month until it becomes a habit. Every Saturday I cook all my food in one batch so that I don't need to think about what I need to eat because there was a time when I was depressed and didn't know anything and I was sitting there thinking I can't be bothered to eat. Or I'm not going to eat, or I really should eat so I'm going to order £50 worth of dominos. Both of them are poor for different reasons, one makes you financially poor and one makes you physically poor. Now I don't really need to have that question in my life anymore because the food is always there.

The more you automate and the more you make things routine, the easier it is to live because you don't have to think. It sounds a bit tragic but the less you think, the easier it is to live. You just do. You put good habits in place so that you don't need to focus on those negative feelings. You can just continue doing things you need to do. The hardest part for somebody who is at the lowest of low is to start implementing those habits and getting out in the first place in finding something to do. That's the hardest part in all honesty.

The third one is Think and Grow Rich by Napoleon Hill, this is for atheist friends. This is one of your classics alongside Dale Carnigie's How to Win Friends and Influence People. On a side note, never meet your heroes because your heroes will always disappoint because they are human too. I met a WWE superstar who actually credits his positive thought through The Secret by Rhonda Byrne. Personally, I feel it's for people who don't have faith who are looking for an answer for their problems. They can't turn to faith because they don't believe in faith so they turn to books like The Secret and there's nothing wrong with that.

One of my colleagues who is very good at what he does, read The Secret and he is the most positive person that I've met.

I digress again.

Everybody talks a lot! "I'm going to change, I'm going to be better, I'm going to go to the gym everyday, I'm going to get that promotion." But nobody ever implements this. You can read all of these books, but if you don't live your life in those ways it's not going to help, likewise a true Christian is somebody who tries to live their lives as close to Jesus as possible, not somebody who goes to church every week and knows the Bible back to front.

So, I met this WWE superstar at a workshop. He said that he recommended reading Think and Grow Rich, and the first chapter is Desire. If you want to be rich you actually really need to want to be rich. It's not just something I wish for. You need to want nothing else in this world.

The second one, faith. You need to want it, and you need to believe that you can get it. Also, an auto suggestion is to always mention that you want it. If you want to be a millionaire it's as simple as saying it every day in the morning looking into your mirror and start a mantra saying 'I'm going to be a millionaire'. It's literally prayer in another form. Self-mantras and then altering other pieces, specialized knowledge, Imagination, organised planning. I mean you have to have actual knowledge of what you are wanting to achieve in order to make your money.

**Imagination,** you need to be able to dream. You need to actually picture yourself in that situation.

**Planning,** you need to know how to get there.

**Persistence,** actually following through, and then you just need to work the power of the mind. but you look at this book, all of it is hope through the power of the mind. This is just faith dressed up in a different book.

It is the most important thing but it is also the hardest thing to have. However, if you have hope that tomorrow is going to be a better day, and you actively seek to do something to make yourself better and be kind to yourself, that's an achievement. **It's having that ability to continue to always see that there is a light at the end of the tunnel because once you don't think there is a light at the end of the tunnel you are gone.**

> **HOPE DOES NOT AND WILL NEVER HAVE AN EXPIRY DATE!**
>
> *Emmanuel Owusu*

# STRESS AND ANXIETY

**Stress causes physical changes in the body designed
to help you take on threats or difficulties.**

'Anxiety' is a word we use to describe feelings of unease, worry and
fear. It incorporates both the emotions and the physical sensations we
might experience when we are worried or nervous about something.
Although we usually find it unpleasant, anxiety is related to the 'fight,
flight or freeze' response – You may notice that your heart pounds,
your breathing quickens, your muscles tense and you start to sweat.- our
normal biological reaction to feeling threatened. Anxiety is considered as
a trait of normal human behaviour however, certain levels of anxiety can
cross a diagnosable threshold. This is usually when it has a pathological
effect on normal human functions.

Once the threat or difficulty passes, these physical effects usually fade.
But if you're constantly stressed, your body stays in a state of high alert
and you may develop stress-related symptoms.

**Symptoms of stress**

Stress can affect how you feel emotionally, mentally and physically, and
also how you behave.

**How you may feel emotionally**

- Overwhelmed
- Irritable and 'wound up'
- Anxious or fearful
- Lacking in self esteem

## How you may feel mentally

- Racing thoughts
- Constant worrying
- Difficulty concentrating
- Difficulty making decisions

## How you may feel physically

- Headaches
- Muscle tension or pain
- Dizziness
- Sleep problems
- Feeling tired all the time
- Eating too much or too little

## How you may behave

- Drinking or smoking more
- Snapping at people
- Avoiding things or people you are having problems with

# Conversation with a Sustainability Associate

**Robert Diamond**, Sustainability Associate, BEng (Hons) MA. MSc, CEng, FCIBSE, CEnv, FEI

### I've read briefly about the WELL Building Standard. Can you tell me a more about what it entails?

The WELL building standard is an American standard that was bought in to help with health and wellbeing in various building types, so in the UK we have BREEAM which undertakes an environmental assessment methodology. We don't have anything else in the UK so the Well standard is really the only standard that primarily focuses on health and wellbeing. It does include other aspects including things like energy and fitness as well as mental health. It is a fairly broad standard but does have particular credits within it that identify certain things that could be done, but the point of the well assessment is to see what is installed, or what is going to be designed into the building.

Because it's an assessment method it doesn't tell you what to do - it scores on what you have done or what is being built into the design so it's not saying you should put in stand/sit desks for example, it says you get points if you have 30% of your desks that are stand/sit. So, it is an assessment methodology that identifies health and wellbeing needs in particular buildings. It's fairly new, 2-3 years old, and it does not from my experience transfer easily into the UK. It's based on American standards and therefore aren't necessarily transferable.

**You've mentioned some of the drawbacks. Does
the BREEAM version have recommendations
which the WELL standards don't?**

So, every 3 or 4 years the BRE update their standard. There's a
consultation document at the moment for the 2018 new construction
system and they are and have included certain aspects of WELL but
because it's only a consultation it's difficult to know what is ultimately
going to happen.

The consultation document is available online for comment and review.
Until it comes out next year we don't really know, but it certainly looks
like the building research establishment who receive the BREEAM
system would include an aspect of WELL and I personally think that
actually we'll end up doing more health and wellbeing aspects as part of
our BREEAM assessments.

I've not heard that they are doing a WELL UK but I know that there
are companies out there who have developed their own, taking bits and
pieces from it, but there's no standard such as BREEAM or LEED so I
think the BRE will be leading the way. That's my guess on next year and
that's the way I think it's going.

**Does the built environment affect the mental
wellbeing and how much so if it does?**

I certainly say yes it does. There's no doubt in my mind and in my
20 years in the industry it certainly does affect mental wellbeing.
I know people that work in very difficult environments and also
expectations about working through lunch and working late, people
eating at their desks not getting fresh air, low ventilation rates, fully
air-conditioned buildings, stress from high level management - you
could go on and on.

Lifestyles today are drive the car to work, sit in front of a computer, go home and sit in front of another computer, go to bed, get up and you're looking at a burnout or a very dull life in my opinion. I don't think we've got it right, I'm generalizing but I think we are miles behind in the UK.

I think the WELL standard is fantastic and is pushing in the right direction but I've been in meetings with clients and spoken about these things and it's been considered "a load of rubbish", that kind of attitude of we are the men we don't take lunch or whatever. That whole old school way of looking at things, so I think we're miles away from good communication, people taking fresh air breaks, thinking about their wellbeing, considering others.

## Is it as simple as it sounds to do the things you have suggested?

I think it's more a state of mind in my opinion. A way of re-looking at what we do and why we do it. The changing state of mind could happen in an instant however it may never happen to certain people. I wonder how much it involves ones' perspective on life and what one has experienced in life. If somebody's had a stroke or a mental breakdown, or suffered from whatever mental illness I think that changes ones' perspective. I think it's very hard when somebody is fairly well and everything is going well to see the other side of the picture, i.e. I worked for my lunch break and I'm alright, but actually many people are not fine.

I think the figures are 1 in 4 people in their lifetime suffer from some kind of mental health illness. That goes to show how prominent it is. To add to that there's also how we work in the modern day, you know the fast responses, the expectation, the mobile phone and email. That has changed radically and that has a big effect on people. The instant response culture. You send an email and you want a response straight away and I don't think that's good for mental health. That's the challenging culture we are living in.

**With regards to the building elements itself is it as simple as I work in an office with a small window, little light, that might affect my mental wellbeing, I should get a bigger window so there is more light?**

No, I don't think it's as simple as that. I think it's complex. It may be an easy answer but I think it is far broader than simple changes. Sure, better lighting, more fresh air will have an effect but it isn't just that. It's the social side, it's how people work with each other it can involve the paints, the plants, air-conditioning.

I'm not saying we shouldn't do the simple things like open up the window but it's far broader than that. It's almost like how we work, even down to working hours and expectations of working hours. I know in some European countries they work less hours and are more productive. There's that whole attitude of you have to be seen in the office from 9-6 or whatever and if you finish the work at 4 and people sit playing on their phones to kill time. Is that healthy to be sitting and not be productive? People work really late but are they really working late or are they there just to be seen to be working to keep the bosses happy? There is a whole culture around money and why we're working to get money - to get things we don't need to impress people we don't like.

Some of the best projects in my mind are when you've got all the stakeholders involved, everybody's aware and everybody is working together as a team. It's very hard to get that team approach. Everybody works in their little boxes, the engineers, the architects, the designers, the project managers. Some forward-thinking companies and clients are doing that but often it's about money and how cheaply you do to make profit and therefore if it's there to make profit you haven't got time to spend discussing or being creative, the fees are just not enough for that.

'It's more a state of mind
A way of re-looking at what we do and
why we do it. The changing state of mind
could happen in an instant however it may
never happen to certain people.'

You send an email and you want a response straight away and I don't think that's good for mental health. That's the challenging culture we are living in.

I know people that work in very difficult environments and also expectations about working through lunch and working late, people eating at their desks not getting fresh air, low ventilation rates, fully air-conditioned buildings, stress from high level management - you could go on and on.

# DOES THE BUILT ENVIRONMENT AFFECT MENTAL HEALTH?

## Emmanuel Owusu, BA(Hons)
## PGdip MSc ACIAT MHFA

## History

The modern history of the connection between the built environment and health can be traced back to the industrial revolution from 1760 to 1840. This was a time when increasing industrialization, immigration, and urbanization resulted in a rapid Increase in the scale of cities and worsened pre-existing problems with sanitation, hygiene and pollution. (LOPEZ, R. 2012). Sanitary surveys were undertaken by reformers who used it to motivate the public and to aid the passing of new laws that eventually resulted in cleaner cities and better public health. By the start of the twentieth century, housing laws and zoning codes affected urban and suburban development. New ideas about the role of architecture in promoting health began to influence the planning and implementation of public health policies.

## Public Perceptions and Assumptions
## Regarding the Built Environment

The modern study of the connection between the built environment and health is a fairly new area of research but it is one that is growing and evolving. The key verdict it that it is not always possible to provide clear links between the two fields. Part of this is a result of the lack of collaboration between researchers, doctors, construction professionals and service users.

A related misconception is that many people assume that rural environments, or living away from the rest of humanity may be some of the healthiest place to live thus leading to a positive mental wellbeing. In actuality, evidence suggests that rural living is less conducive to good health than urban living despite of the quitter surrounding, scenic views, lack of overcrowding. The finding of the research that proves this hypothesis contradicts the widely believed rationale that moving to the suburbs provides healthier environment.

## What is the built environment?

According to (LOPEZ, R. 2012), the term 'built environment' refers to all the many ways humanity builds or manipulates the world around it. The health effects of the built environment happen on multiple scales, including houses, streets, neighbourhoods, metropolitan areas, regions, nations, and beyond. The built environment provides the framework for how daily lives are conducted, influences health across life spans, and represents important pathways through which individuals come into contact with many health risks.

To different people, the term 'environment' is very broad and can mean many things. Even researchers and scientist from different disciplines varying definitions of what constitute the environment. Lopez further explains that the environment can be divided into three broad spheres: the physical, social, and built environments. The physical environment constitutes all the varying features that are part of mainstream environmental literature such as: forests, prairies, watersheds, plants, animals, and so on. It also includes the factors that are of concern to classic environmental health: air and water pollutants, radiation hazards, and so forth.

On the other hand, the social environment is more concerned with many features which result from or are part human interaction with each other. These include the role of race in society, politics, distribution of income and other similar factors. Large body of research exist which shows that the social environment can have profound impacts on health. For instance, even though race is a social rather than a biological construct, the perception of an individual's race can have important lifelong impacts on mental wellbeing. Race itself can influence income and wealth, which in turn can then lead to an individual's ability to live near parks and other environmental amenities. Additionally, It may place limitations to certain neighbourhoods, thus affecting an individual's exposure to hazardous wastes or influencing access to nutritious food.

Lastly, the built environment itself consists of a conglomerate of many features that have been constructed by humanity. These include many things such as how rooms are laid out, the construction of homes, the various land uses in a neighbourhood, planning laws which affect the structure of neighbourhoods and metropolitan areas (Lopez, R 2012).

## Daylighting and wellbeing

Employers and researchers face tougher challenges to design working environments that can best meet the needs of 21st century workers to ensure maximum levels of well-being and thus performance. Existing research documents provides good evidence of a connection between lighting, work performance and well-being in the workplace. Studies shows that lighting can be one of the key contributing factors that combine to create a healthy work environment which in turn helps promote employee engagement and productivity. Providing 'positive' levels of lighting can be important in employers attracting and retaining professional workers.

In regard to how the lighting in the various offices affect them, some of the employees at a company I surveyed commented:

- *'Having a window to look out of is both relaxing and helpful for work.'*
- *'Lighting does impact well-being, there is not enough natural daylight in this office'*

- *'I prefer to use my desk light'*
- *'I would prefer to be nearer a window for more natural daylight'*
- *'There's very little ambient light'*
- *'I value having natural lighting, there are factors that definitely improve my mood. Also, the ability to open a window gives you a feeling of control over your environment.'*

Investing in a variety of workplace lighting should be high on the agenda of employers as a means to develop work environments that support well-being and performance. This can lead to a reduction in the likelihood of employee stress, sickness and absenteeism.

The challenge employers face is that certain groups of employees might prefer brighter lighting environments whilst others might not. Therefore, perhaps a way of arranging a layout that could be based on the preferences of employee groups in relation to lighting might be a possible solution. It's a good idea to consider a seating arrangement based on worker's lighting preference. This could boost mood and well-being which in turn can increase worker's productivity and performance.

Although the area of lighting is one of the more researched in the factors that affect well-being, there is still a need for a more focus capturing and measuring the impact of lighting on employee well-being and performance, in order to build an evidence base to support workplace initiatives.

## Summary

Similar to the notion that there is no single factor that causes an individual to experience mental illness, I believe that there is no single design solution that can lead to an improvement in one's mental health. There needs to be a holistic approach where many factors work together to have a positive impact. Whilst there is research that support the belief that a better designed built environment can lead to a better mental health, this is not a singular element. Additionally, it must be stated that sometimes no matter how well designed the built environment is, it cannot lead to an improvement in one's wellbeing. This often depends on the cause of the illness and/or the severity of the individual's deterioration of their mental state.

There is a general consensus with those that work in the built environment that the built environment does indeed affect mental health because it can affect one's state of wellbeing.

As a simple recommendation, in order to produce a design that is conducive to improving one's mental health, a combination of design features need to be applied to attain a result;

Providing just one design or a limited performance issue will not necessarily improve wellbeing. A flexibility in the design such as offering open plan and private offices can help. Additionally, providing the ability for the individual to change their environment gives them freedom, choice and control. These can be in the form of providing dimmable lighting, windows that can open to allow certain amounts of light during different times in the day can also lead to a positive mental health. An important factor which wasn't explored was designing the layout in such a way that the employees can easily communicate with one another and ask for help if they are having difficulties with tasks thus reducing stress.

7

Good practice in the design of a space can return the following:

- **Increased concentration**
- **Reduced eye strain & healthy sleeping cycle**
- **Reduce stress and increased resilience**
- **Increased creativity and focus**
- **Enhanced group identity and emotional support**
- **Increased concentration, reduced headaches**

Following the results of my research, the key recommendation is for designers to approach how we design the office space in a holistic manner. They should provide a wide range of design solutions. They should understand that whilst the good design of the building itself can have a positive effect on mental health, the most significant influence is the ethos of the company and how business is conducted. Employees offering to help one another and speaking respectfully and supporting one another can have a more positive impact on a worker's mental health than the design of the building itself.

Wellbeing cannot be added to a person but It can be 'taken away' by the (built) environment and lifestyle that surrounds that person. Therefore, as professionals, let us design our office buildings so that it does not take away the wellbeing to a person.

# Psychosis

## Definition and Symptoms

Psychosis is a mental health problem that causes people to perceive or interpret things differently from those around them. This might involve hallucinations or delusions.

The two main symptoms of psychosis are:

**Hallucinations** – where a person hears, sees and, in some cases, feels, smells or tastes things that aren't there; a common hallucination is hearing voices.

**Delusions** – where a person has strong beliefs that aren't shared by others; a common delusion is someone believing there is a conspiracy to harm them.

The combination of hallucinations and delusional thinking can cause severe distress and a change in behaviour.

Experiencing the symptoms of psychosis is often referred to as having a psychotic episode.

## Causes of psychosis

It's sometimes possible to identify the cause of psychosis as a specific mental health condition, such as:

**schizophrenia** – a condition that causes a range of psychological symptoms, including hallucinations and delusions.

**bipolar disorder** – a mental health condition that affects mood; a person with bipolar disorder can have episodes of low mood (depression) and highs or elated mood (mania).

**severe depression** – some people with depression also have symptoms of psychosis when they're very depressed.

Psychosis can also be triggered by:

a traumatic experience
stress
drug misuse
alcohol misuse
side effects of prescribed medication
a physical condition – such as a brain tumour

How often a psychotic episode occurs and how long it lasts can depend on the underlying cause.

# Conversation with a Psychiatric Epidemiologist

Dr. James Kirkbride,
BA, MSc, PHD

*Reader in Epidemiology, Division of Psychiatry, Faculty of Brain Sciences, University College London*

## What is your role within mental health?

I am a psychiatric epidemiologist, so my training is in epidemiology, originally in geography so I come from a social science background so I am not a clinician or psychiatrist. I've had no medical training but I have worked in academic psychiatry departments at universities for over 15 years now so I have an understanding of mental health problems from having worked there and having done my PHD in this field. My background is in epidemiology so I'm interested in population health and how diseases and disorders vary between different populations, and within populations between different groups. We usually use large data sets to compare risk in different groups of people.

So that's my background. I've got a particular interest in spatial patterns in health, which led me to this idea (which many others before me have also had!) that psychosis might be environmental, that there may be some factors in our environment that aren't good for our mental health. Things like living in a highly-deprived area or stressful neighbourhoods. During my research it became apparent that one of the biggest topics in this area is migration and ethnicity, and that not just the Black community in the UK, but migrants all over the world tend to experience this phenomenon of higher rates of psychosis and that risk persists into the children often and into their children's children as far as we can tell. I'm really interested in 2 things, the urban environment and the social environment and how migration and ethnicity play into that risk as well.

A friend pointed out that a few years ago speaking in a public place, about mental health would be unthinkable.

I think that's a really interesting change in our culture that we've witnessed and it's great. That's come about for so many reasons. Partly it's coming from the bottom up, people are less afraid to talk about their mental health problems and that's through things like social media where you have outlets for being able to talk about things, but partly it's coming from the top as well, from all the work, especially by the Liberal democrats in the last government, to get mental health on the agenda when they were in coalition with the Tories. Remarkably at least the dialogue about that has stayed since, though sadly not necessarily the investment, which I think is still way off what it should be, but the dialogue about mental health from high-up politically has helped a lot.

People are much more willing to talk about it, their own issues and just acknowledge it as a whole. I think that's great. There is still a long way to go for example, recently I published a study based in East Anglia and we spent 5 years collecting data on all the people who had been to early intervention services for their first episode of psychosis.

The study wanted to address lots of important questions. For example, we don't know very much about the incidence of schizophrenia and other psychotic disorders as they are in rural communities, so we partly set up the study for that purpose. Included in that were also questions about whether some ethnic minority groups have an increased risk of psychosis in rural areas.

You'll be aware that that's higher in the Black African and Black Caribbean communities in this country, and in other countries like the Moroccan communities in the Netherlands etc., but we didn't know whether that same phenomenon existed in more rural areas where ethnic minority groups are often even smaller in terms of their overall proportion of the population. So, we set it up to investigate that and we found that just like in urban areas, ethnic minority groups still had a raised rate of psychosis and that was strongest again for the Black African and Black Caribbean groups. We tried to see whether that was explained by basic alternate explanations, like maybe different age profiles of that group compared to the white group, different sex profiles or different socio-economic profiles.

There was some explanation that it was partly that those group on average had lower social economic positions, but that didn't explain the entire risk. We published this study in a journal called Schizophrenia Bulletin and it got a bit of press, it got covered by a good article in The Guardian and then it was picked up by The Voice and they published a story on it saying how the study was totally wrong, how it was all down to racist stereotyping and prejudices of the researchers, and of the psychiatry community, who they said are more likely to over diagnose people from ethnic minority backgrounds. I think there was a case to be made that that was a legitimate possibility, but the article in The Voice completely dismissed any possibility that the study could have produced a genuine result, that actually in the UK we might see that there are massive mental health inequalities for psychosis for people from minority ethnic groups.

It dismissed that as an idea altogether without considering that it might be true, and I was really disappointed by that, because in all these ways we've opened up about mental health, and how people are more willing to talk about mental health, and that includes different communities talking about their mental health problems. Even if you look on the Voice website there are loads of really good articles about people opening up about their experiences with depression and anxiety disorders, but when it came to psychosis, which is one of the most stigmatized, the message is still that this couldn't be true, that it had to be down to something else. In that instant I felt like we made very little progress about tackling the stigma around psychosis.

## You mentioned a link between the built environment and psychosis. What have you found in your research?

I think the research on the built-in environment and psychosis and in general mental health more broadly is massively under researched. There is fairly limited evidence that the built-in environment itself has a direct connection to psychosis risk. It's not that it doesn't, it's just that we don't know, and it needs testing. Where we do see more evidence is for the social environment and in particular, areas with higher population densities, areas with higher rates of deprivation and higher rates of economic inequality seem to have these higher rates of disorder.

One could theorise that that might be due to the stresses that emerge when you are living in areas where you're constantly exposed to limited opportunity. So you might come from a low socio-economic background or you might come from a rough or deprived area and that might be stressful in itself, particularly when you factor inequality on top of that. If you're then forced to make comparisons between your socio-economic position and that of people around you. South London is quite a good example, when you're walking down 2 different kinds of estates in the same street. One estate is a higher rise building and you literally turn the corner and you are in a beautiful park estate where the houses cost 3 million pounds each and they're virtually on the same street. When you're forced either consciously or subconsciously to be exposed to that type environment and make comparisons maybe that can be quite stressful.

Then population density on top of that is another form of stress if you think about overcrowding and that kind of thing. That might be related to your chance at developing psychosis, so from a very broad level that's how we tend to think about it. The built-in environment of course can factor into that, and that's what we don't know. We know that population density is really strongly associated to psychosis risk and that extends to where you're born, so if you're born in a more urban environment your risk of psychosis is higher 25 years later, so that link does exist.

If that's a causal link then can we design better environments with, for example, more low-density housing that might improve social conditions; it may not be the housing itself that's the problem, but it might be that low-density housing fosters different types of community cohesion, different types of integration with other people, so it's how the built-in environment connects us to the social which I think is the more relevant part.

Last year I was asked to give a talk to a consultancy firm called Arup, and they basically have a session where they bring in 30 of their brightest consultants and they have a theme for the session. Last year's theme was on people and society. Part of it was that they wanted to know how they could design better buildings for mental health. I thought that it was fantastic because it is on people's agenda and people are thinking less in terms of insulation and so on, which nowadays are taken for granted and what's not is how we build better environments for our mental health and for our physical health as well. I'm glad that's coming up as an agenda item.

## We have a framework for dementia and physical disability, can we create a design framework for mental health? How can it be done?

As an epidemiologist, my job is to identify who is at risk of developing a disorder in the population, so part of my job is talking is discovering who these most people are. So if we knew that most people suffering from depression favoured buildings that were lighter or that had better lighting design, we can do something about that. We recognise that it wouldn't fit everybody, but it's fitting the majority or the highest risk group, and it's about making those kind of choices as to how to respond to our environment.

You can never necessarily get everything right for everybody because of that variability, but you can get the majority which is probably more important. Whether you measure the majority as the number of people or the number of high risk people which might lead to a slightly different answer which you would need to do research. My second point on that is as an academic, the starting point for all of this is evidence. We need evidence that it works. A mental health building code would be the most amazing thing ever wouldn't it? The same way if we could recognise that buildings needed ramp access, wheelchair friendly things if we had something similar with mental health it would be a wonderful place.

We need to say this is what works and this is what doesn't work for the majority of people. Only then can we redesign buildings effectively, because if you don't have that leadership from evidence you can't advise Arup or whoever it is to do things because if we don't know that something will work then ultimately it is not going to be beneficial for the people living there and that's what matters.

In regards to evidence, is it because there is a lack of evidence or a lack of research? How do we improve that?

The evidence about the built environment and mental health is missing. It's not that it's not there it's just that we haven't tested it properly. You will read a lot about this topic in the general press, and some academic forums, but when you drill down to the evidence it's simply not good enough. This area is under-funded and I think the solution is for people, not just people like me, but for people to actually start applying our brains and find a path to address this, because the reason it attracts public attention, or increasing public attention is because intuitively it makes sense. But we need the science to support or refute that.

The built-in environment should have an effect on how we feel, if it's a good design then we feel great about it, and if we see the design is ugly and horrific we will feel less good about it. It would seem legitimate that from a theoretical prospective that could happen we just need the studies to do that and that requires investment, and creative thinking from the academics to design the right type of study. A lot of studies are often small or using convenient samples, or badly tested or badly designed. What we need is some gold standard evidence that funders also believe in.

I think part of the problem is slippery concept like how you actually measure, objectively measure good or bad design is a difficult thing to do. When you're talking about heart disease and smoking and drinking it's very easy to measure how many cigarettes you take etc, it's harder to say what is the quantitative feeling I get from this building outside, so that's difficult. I think funders are sometimes reluctant to fund the social side because it's a slippery construct but that's our best challenge we need to meet.

## From your studies and experience how has that stigma linked to mental health?

There has been an enormous amount of stigma with mental health particularly with Psychosis. It's a challenge that we face. It works in two ways as far as I can see it, maybe more. One is that the stigma anyone can experience. We broaden out that stigma concept, we can think of things like bullying and discrimination for any kind of reason and we know that those are associated as a risk factor for mental health problems. They increase your risk of mental health and I think that's quite established.

Then there is the stigma once you have a mental health disorder, and presumably they are not unrelated, they are circular. So if some kind of stigma, harassment or discrimination has increased your risk and if that stigma is made worse because you have a mental health disorder then that can perpetuate worse outcomes for you going forward. So there's that kind of stigma, the causal relationship between stigma and mental health, and then the consequential relationship of having a mental health disorder which leads to worse outcomes maybe as a result of increased stigma.

Then there is the other kind of stigma, the institutional stigma that people might go up against when they have a mental health problem in the NHS. We know for example that people with mental health problems in general tend to get worse physical care with the NHS because when you are presented with depression, anxiety, psychosis and often the first thing that's done is to look at your mental health but forget about your physical health needs as well.

That's gotten better for sure. Now there's physical health checks when you go to an early intervention service, or at least there should be. That is getting better but stigma can apply at that institutional level where people with mental health problems might get worse, physical health treatment for example somehow because the disorder obscures the clinician from treating people appropriately and treating people equally.

**Following from that, how can we eradicate the stigma. Is it possible to eradicate it?**

Aids is a good example, where there was a huge problem with it and they had no answer at the time when it emerged in the early 80s. There was no cure or prevention. There was no treatment initially which of course creates an enormous amount of fear and from fear comes ignorance, stigma and prejudice. You can see a similar trajectory with mental health problems. The answer as you said with aids was to do more research, put more investment in and understand the disease process, understand how to combat it, understand how to treat people with Aids and HIV, and of course now people with HIV enjoy good life expectancies on average. That has to help with the stigma, the public now understands how HIV is transmitted and the risks to take.

So I think to reduce the stigma with mental health we need to apply similar principles where we invest in the disorders in terms of understand where they come from, how they're caused, and that a better understanding and convergence of ideas about how mental health problems arise will destigmatise them for the public. I mean there has even been ideas where you can somehow catch depression or psychosis from somebody, and I think that's very old fashioned now, I don't think many reasonably educated people will think that. There's still a stigma, there's still a misunderstanding about it so I think that's helped.

The question about whether we can completely eradicate the stigma? I believe we can't. As with anything in society there are always people who are less ignorant or more ignorant. That applies to any part of society. There's always people who have a fixed view of something and can never change it. So I think it is impossible to eradicate but something we can certainly minimise and do something about.

**I know you are not a clinician or a medical doctor, but what advice would you give to someone who is or knows someone dealing with mental health?**

Working with mental health professionals a lot, I think the advice we always give is to approach your GP as your first point of call. I think they are under used, overused in every single way possible, but they are under used in terms of mental health as a gateway into mental health services. People have fears about going to their GP in terms of anything from a flu symptom to a bad back, to mental health problems. We need to not be afraid to do that and to talk to our GPs about our mental health problems and it might be difficult for some people to do that but then there's opportunities hopefully to talk to family or friends in confidence and they might suggest other routes, but usually the first point of call is to speak to a health care professional or at least charity services available such as helplines to get some advice from somebody who is impartial.

From a personal perspective just talking to someone who is impartial is the most amazing thing in the world. To be able to talk to someone without them judging your issues, you can rationalise them in a way that is impossible to do sometimes with family or friends. Although they want to be supportive, their support isn't always channeled in the right way or it doesn't express itself in the right way. Talking to someone impartial, it's enormously helpful because they are not judgmental, they've seen it before, they know what they are talking about and they can advise you and help you.

# CONVERSATION WITH SENIOR UNIVERSITY TEACHER

**Satwinder Samra, RIBA**
Director Collaborative Practice
Senior University Teacher, Sheffield University
MArch Admissions Tutor

## Who are you? What do you do?

I am an Architect, Educator, Dengineer and Father. After graduating with a first class honours and distinction from Sheffield University, I was lucky to be able to start my architectural career with Urban Splash working on leading regeneration projects. After this I joined Proctor Matthews Architects focusing on social housing. I then returned to the urban North, founding Sauce Architecture. I am currently Director of Collaborative Practice and Senior University Teacher at the University of Sheffield School of Architecture and consultant to OSLA an international architecture practice. I am a Designer for 'The Dengineers' on CBBC with Tony Broomhead where we promote architecture to a younger audience. I am also a Trustee of S1 Artspace and an RIBA Role Model to promote diversity in Architecture.

## What are the factors causing mental ill health amongst architecture students?

Architecture is a fascinating, varied and highly challenging yet rewarding discipline. The education can be long, arduous and expensive. Students assume it will take 7 years to qualify but on average for many its takes longer! Some take more years out to build experience and finances before returning to Part 2. The design process itself although highly rewarding can at times be difficult to negotiate and mentally taxing.

Reflecting on my early years as a student of Architecture, I remember that the studio based design projects often seemed confusing, overwhelming and difficult. With personal hindsight and the experience gained from teaching many cohorts of students in different institutions, I have realized that this is not an uncommon experience. For some students this can lead to anxiety, doubting one's own ability and that awful feeling that you are on the wrong path.

Positive Grey is a phrase I often use to describe and highlight the part of the design process that exists part way through the project. All designers acknowledge the importance of creativity during the inception, development and resolution of a project. Design is often about dealing with unknowns. This often occurs in the middle of a project. This middle I refer to as the Positive Grey.

This is something that students need to acknowledge, accept and capture. By being comfortable with uncertainty and doubt they will not only enjoy the project more but also produce better, richer and more diverse work.

Ultimately if we embrace this as part of the process and not as a failing of the student we could go along way to alleviating some of the pressures that individuals face.

## Can you comment whether this is higher than students studying other subject?

There is more awareness and discussion around mental health and well being which is a good thing. However I feel that students are probably feeling more pressure and anxiety due to a number of factors: higher fees, pressure to attain and also future career opportunities. I think this is magnified in architecture given the length of courses and lower salaries commanded by architects when they finally enter the profession. Raising awareness is really important. The work that (ABS) Architects Benevolent Society is developing in this area is invaluable.

## Why did you decide to become an educator?

I've always have been involved in education. During my first job with Urban Splash I taught a day a week at Liverpool John Moores and at Manchester School of Architecture. Jonathan Falkingham and Tom Bloxham headed Urban Splash up; they were really supportive and encouraged me to teach whilst working in practice. I also taught at Brighton during my next job with Proctor Matthews in London, again the directors encouraged teaching whilst practising at the same time.

After my time in London I had the chance to travel so I left my job and spent some time in Canada and America. This gave me the chance to reflect and consider what to do next. On my return I didn't want to go back into conventional practice, so I approached my former tutor Russell Light who offered me some teaching work at Sheffield University School of Architecture. I also teamed up with Daniel Jary to set up Sauce Architecture.

Looking back now, I think both were a way of re- navigating my architectural career and allowing myself to build upon my previous experiences. I've been fortunate to lead both Y3 BA Architecture and the MArch at the Sheffield School. This has given me the chance to work with, encourage and develop over 1500 students. Being an educator offers an opportunity to share my passion not only for the subject but also support students to become rounded, agile, happy people.

## What are some of the ideas/solutions we can implement in our architecture schools to improve students' mental wellbeing?

- **No more lone rangers/myth of** the genius More teamwork and collaboration in all aspects of architectural education needs to be expanded and encouraged. Being part of a team in the learning process encourages mutual support and communication, this goes against the idea of the lone ranger/lone genius model that perpetuates much of architectural education but in reality promotes isolation.

-**Not Open All hours Schools should not be open 24hours a day.** Being open around the clock sends out a signal that to produce the best work you should be working all the time as opposed to teaching students to work efficiently and have a balance their lives. Our studios are not open 24 hours a day. I actively encourage our students to engage in a diverse, varied range of activities. I truly believe that the best work is produced when people have chance to stop, reflect and recharge.

**Positive Grey** - It's ok to be comfortable with uncertainty and doubt during the design process. Only then will students not only enjoy the project more but also produce better, richer and more diverse work. Ultimately having greater awareness and understanding of the process of design can and should lead to calmer, essentially happier students who are less stressed and anxious.

**Learning as a positive experience.** We need to remember that schools of architecture are places for learning. Students need to feel safe and supported as they navigate the complexity of design projects whilst also facing escalating financial pressures.

## Does stigma about mental health exist in architectural education?

Maybe, but I think It's getting better, given that many Universities have good pastoral support. Mental health is being openly discussed more often. In my MArch studio we are exploring mental health and wellbeing not only in the studio projects but also in the students own everyday experiences.

## What support is available to your students regarding mental health?

We offer pastoral care and support. We are also developing new structures including mentoring/buddy groups where more senior students are available to nurture, listen and be there for those who are new to architecture school. There has also been a recent interest from my students who are actively writing about mental health and wellbeing in their MArch Dissertations. Recently David Hodgson, Ashley Mayes and Josh Brookes have produced some exceptional research, which we are now using to change some of our practices.

### Any comment about the Critique / Review process in architecture school?

Many problems and attitudes in the profession stem from educational platform of the crit. Here students' present work to visiting critics who need to be questioning and inquisitive but can often be overbearing and aggressive in their review of the work presented. It is no surprise then that the student adopts a defensive approach in an attempt to 'protect' their work.

The rituals and structures of the 'Crit' are fundamentally flawed. The adversarial and confrontational nature that manifests itself within this process needs an overhaul. Compromise and resolution aren't often encouraged. Let's remember this is a learning environment not a stage for self-centered critics to pass judgement and revel in the spectacle of their own knowledge using the students' work as a backdrop.

Many years ago we made a conscious decision and abandoned the Crit as a term in favour of the Review as this signifies a collective and combined approach between students, tutors and guest reviewers.

At the Sheffield School we encourage dialogue and participation in our reviews. Students are expected to comment and reflect on each other's work through actively taking part in the review. Tutors are actively encouraged to listen, support, nurture and teach!

Obviously the student needs to develop the ability to advocate and promote their work but this should be with support and direction in a positive way. The reviewer has a responsibility to act as an educator and mentor in the process. In doing, so I believe we may foster a generation of less arrogant, more open and inclusive designers who may be able to respond to the challenges of our time.

## 9. What does hope mean to you? How can hope be related to education and mental health?

It's all about being optimistic. Enjoying the process of design and revealing not only the potential of the project but also your own potential and the potential of others. There are no correct answers, nothing is original. There are just opportunities. Let's nurture and celebrate the production of ideas and projects, supporting the next generation to truly believe in themselves.

# CONVERSATION WITH A
# SPEAKER AND TRAINER

Joseph Amoah, BSc

## Do you know anyone who has experienced mental ill health?

Yes. In the early stages of my life, I was not familiar with the concept of mental health. Now that I am older and look back, I recognise that it was a case that was related to mental illness. There have been people around me that I have engaged with when looking back, I discovered that they suffered with various forms of mental ill health largely behave of their behaviour and certain traits. I found this strange and was unsure about what I should do. I found the behaviour peculiar because of the paranoia and anxiety that they expressed.

## Why do you think men find it more difficult to speak about mental health and general health issues?

First and foremost, I believe that as men, this has to do with our society. It is not culturally acceptable for a man to start expressing that they are unhappy. There are certain type of emotions which are more acceptable to express such as rage and anger. These are contrary to things we perceive as being 'soft'. His has a big impact in terms of how men deal with the subject. As an example, if a man is feeling sad, this might transpire in the form of rage which is perceived as an 'alpha male' type of emotion.

## Contrast with African cultural views and western attitudes to mental health.

I believe that there are some distinct differences. Having been born and grown up in Ghana, West Africa, I found that men were perceived as the bread winners who have to show a strong hand of strength. On the other hand, women are more of the nurturing type who are expected to remain at home. Be it your father, uncle or a significant male man, they are seen as the strong figure. In my personal experience, I did not find men expressing their feelings to be something that is common. It is not easy to men in that culture to admit that they may be struggling with mental health challenges. This is the African culture that I experienced growing up.

The western culture is similar but there are noticeable differences. The expectation is, if you are a man, you should be a 'manly man' however, if you do not portray that, you can be classified as a 'girlie man'. With that notion, if some men do not act in the supposedly 'manly' manner, they can be labelled as being 'fruity'.

With the African culture, you are either a 'Manly man' or you are not whereas with the Western culture, there is more of a spectrum. However, this still works in a way that makes men less expressive about their emotions. This is a big issue when it comes to mental health because, as a man, you are still trying to deny any aspect of negative, somewhat depressive feelings. In denying that, it is difficult to then address it and seek help.

## How do we smash the stigma and change the perceptions surrounding mental health?

Specifically for men, there has to be an embrace how we feel. This includes positive and negative emotions. On an individual level, you must be honest with what is happening. This does not make you weaker. As human beings, we all have emotions. Mental health is something that if you do not take care of, it can have a significant negative consequences.

In general, there has to be an embrace of awareness. The reason why I did not understand the behaviours is because there was not enough information about the subject. People do not talk about it. It was not in the media. Thankfully now, this is improving but it is nowhere near the level I believe it should be at. People do not know how to relate to someone who has mental health issues. These people themselves, feel like an outcast. Therefore, there has to be more information available.

**What does hope mean to you? How can this be related to mental health?**

When we speak of hope in this context, it can be challenging. **HOPE IS WHAT KEEPS US ALIVE!** Without hope, there is no point living. For me, hope is two letter: 'E' 'E'. This stands for eager expectations. This is something that will come to past but may not necessarily be in the present. There is hope even if you suffer from mental health issues. **As long as you are alive, you must expect positive things to happen.** This is in spite of doctors giving negative medical reports. **When hope is lost, it can be dangerous.** We must always maintain a sense of personal hope. If you suffer from mental ill health or know someone who does, maintaining hope can help them get better.

HOPE IS WHAT KEEPS US ALIVE!

As long as you are alive, you
MUST expect positive things to happen.

**When hope is lost,
it can be dangerous**

# Conversation with a National Professional Advisor in Forensic Mental Health National at Care Quality Commission

Paul Gilluley,

*Opera loving, ballroom dancing psychiatrist
who always sees the glass half full!.*

**What's your association with mental health? Have you directly experienced or know anyone/have encountered anyone with a mental health issue?**

I had personal experience of mental health from a very early age. My mother died when I was 18 months old and we went to live with my paternal grandparents. At that time my great grandmother was also at home and suffering from Alzheimers dementia. She was unable to recognise my grandmother as her daughter and used to tell me she was keeping her in the housed against her will and that her daughter had run off with a sailor. She was often telling us bizarre stories. My grandfather also suffered from multi infarct dementia and by the time I was a toddler he was also blind and deaf. I remember it as a very busy household, but it was also one where I felt very loved and cared for.

**What are some of the medical / clinical methods to managing/improving our mental health?**

Mental health is complex to manage/ improve mental health you cannot just take as medical approach. I was always taught a medico/ psycho/ social approach to address any mental health issues. Medical tends to be thought of as medication and has a biochemical basis to the theory behind use of medication for mental health issues. Psychological allows use of talking therapies of different types to be used. Social emphasises the needs for social change to allow mental health to be managed or improved.

## Why do you think suicide rates amongst men is higher than women?

It is obvious but men are different from women and as a result have different needs. Men traditionally are not great talkers about emotional issues. This also has a cultural mind set too of men being strong and protectors of their family. To admit any weakness would be seem as a fault. They therefore are more likely to store things up and less likely to talk things through with friends.

## Why do you think men do not like to discuss the topic of mental health?

Talking about mental health in general has been difficult until relatively recently. Shutting people with mental health problems away in asylums did not happen that long ago. People wanted to see those with mental health problems as different from themselves and tended to keep them at arms length. Prominent people talking about their issues with mental health is a recent phenomenon. Getting men to talk openly about emotional issues may take a bit longer.

## Are men more susceptible to have mental health issues than women?

As mentioned above men are different from women so their needs are different. How they present with mental health problems are also different. Some mental health issues are more common in men than women and in others it is the other way about.

## From your experience what are some of the common causes that can lead to a mental health issue?

There are so many factors that need to be taken into consideration that I am not sure there is a simple answer. Your genetic make-up and your personality characteristics need to be taken into consideration. As a result of this some may have lower or higher thresholds for developing mental health problems. We then have to take into consideration the social world you are exposed to. This includes relationships (both good and bad) As well as experience (again both good and bad). This mix is different and specific for each individual person.

## Why is there a stigma regarding mental health? Where does this come from?

We try to prevent ourselves from identifying with mental health problems as we are concerned that this shows some weakness within us.

## Can the stigma be eradicated in its entirety?

Stigma will never go away and to think it is gone would be a problem in itself.

## What are some of the most useful ways we can address the stigma and change it?

Acknowledging difference in others and embracing that difference would be a start.

## From your experience Is/are there certain demographic(s) of people who are more prone to having mental health issues?

We have data to suggest that more young black men are detained under the mental health act and also detained in secure mental health hospitals. The reason for this are multifactorial and we are doing work at the minute to understand this better. This is useful, but we also need to be proactive and look at ways we can prevent this from continuing to happen in the future.

## Why have the rates of mental health issues risen so much over the years?

Some of this is due to better identification. In the past many lived in the community without any diagnosis of mental health issues. Access to services is now much wider.

## How do you maintain a positive mental health?

I am acutely aware of trying to maintain positive mental health. Keeping a work life balance is important for me. I struggle with this at times although I acknowledge I need time to chill with come space to myself. Also remembering my mother's advice of all things in moderation. I have never been great at that.

## What does hope mean to you? How can the notion be associated with mental health?

Hope is extremely important and when in crisis it can be very easy (and dangerous) to lose hope. For some people with mental health issues there are times when they are unable to hold onto hope. It is my opinion that at these times it is important that we as mental health clinicians hold onto that hope for them. When they are ready to take it back we need to support them.

## What advice would you give to someone experiencing mental ill health?

Two things that have been said already **"never lose hope"** and **"always talk it through"** there will always be someone there to listen.

*Also remembering my mother's advice*
*of 'all things in moderation.'*

*"never lose hope" and "always talk it through"*
*there will always be someone there to listen.*

# LOOK AFTER YOUR BODY: CONVERSATION WITH A PERSONAL TRAINER

Bola Cole, Personal Trainer
(The Gym Group)

As part of my recovery, my care coordinator and GP encouraged me to join my local gym and to take part in Badminton and Cycling therapy classes aimed at improving my physical health. They explained that improving my physical condition and taking part in active sports would have a significant benefit on my mental wellbeing aiding my recovery. To this end, I signed up to sessions with a personal trainer who understood this notion of the benefit to the mind when the body is in a healthy state. I encouraged him to share some of his wealth of knowledge about how looking after the body can benefit the mind.

*Bola Cole (Personal Trainer) I personally believe that there is a direct and clear link between how the mind and body work. In psychology and even in philosophy there has been an ongoing debate whether this is true. For instance, is the body considered to simply be an extension of the mind or is the mind a part of the body? I do take the view that there is definitely a link between the two. When I train my clients, I intentionally ask them to think about the specific exercise that they're doing, to think about the action and to think about initiating that muscle movement. I find that this results in a better work out.*

*To do any action, the brain sends an impulse to the specific muscles. It relays messages to the core muscle group. Having this in mind, I wouldn't say it makes the work out easier but rather more effective. Exercise is amazing! As you exercise, your brain releases 'feel good hormones' such as serotonin and dopamine. Take an example when you are stressed, the body reacts by releasing stress hormones. In that moment, the body is responding to the stresses and reacts in a variety of ways; for example, your heart rate might* increase. This can be linked to a 'flight or fight' response showing that there is certainly a link between the mind and the body. These stresses can be very damaging to the body. If your body is constantly going through such heights, it can have an impact on your mental health. You seem to find that when a lot of people have gone through stressful situations, their mental wellbeing can start to slowly deteriorate and this is common.

I have worked at a few leisure centres where they have something called 'Referrals'. This is where GP's and doctors have referred people who may have a mental health issue to exercise at the centre as an aid to improve their wellbeing. I've known people with depression having been referred to the leisure centre. As they work out, the feel good hormones are released which in turn helps to reduce stress. Additionally, this can make the body and the mind less susceptible to illnesses. I believe that a well put together exercise program can be a standalone treatment for some mental illnesses e.g. depression.

Marcus Tullius Cicero who was a Roman philosopher amongst many things famously said that **"It is exercise alone that supports the spirits, and keeps the mind in vigor"**. So even before the advent of modern medicine, there was an understanding that predated all of the modern medicinal solutions as to how to have a vigorous mind. There was an understanding and an awareness that one's physical and mental health are directly linked.

Going back to the example I said regarding the body being in a stressful 'fight or flight' zone, that response doesn't just last in that moment. Even after the stimulus has passed, there is still residue where the stress hormones released by the body is still effective. This principle is the same when you exercise. The contrasting feel good hormone that is released when you exercise doesn't simply stop as soon as the exercise is over. It continues to have very positive effect throughout the day.

A person might get into an argument with someone and you hear people advise them to 'walk it off' or to 'go punch some bags.' All these are forms of exercise which results in the person usually feeling destressed and often less angry. There has been much research conducted with different groups of people where one group exercises frequently and the other group doesn't. It's been documented that the group that exercise often usually are healthier, not just physically but also mentally. Even when we observe people's memory, research has proven an increase in cognitive function due to exercise.

Many things happen when you work out. Each action and movement has a profound effect on the body at a deeper level which in turn benefits the mind. This effect can have a positive effect in your daily life. For some people, having an hour of their day where they are working out is the highlight because they are not focusing on the stresses in their lives during that period.

One of the issues when someone is going through depression is a negative self-worth and self-esteem. One of the benefits of exercise is that the individual makes a conscious effort to better themselves. This in turn often leads to the individual having a positive self-perception and self-value. This is why I believe a good exercise program can be a good alternative to medication when dealing with some mental health illnesses.

# CONVERSATION WITH A FOOTBALLER

Nana Boakye Yiadom

**Being a professional sportsman, how do you think exercise can help with physical and mental health.**

In terms of physical health, being in the right space physical and being as fit as possible will have an impact mentally. For instance, if I am in peak physical condition, this will affect what I do in terms of the small tasks. In my head, I will feel confident because I feel good physically. This will mean that I will have a mentally outlook, not just about football but about myself as a human being. Physical and mental health go hand in hand. If i am in a good physical condition I can perform at an optimum level mentally.

**Having progressed through an elite English football academy system at a young age, were you trained to deal with disappointment?**

I was at West Ham United F.C from the age of thirteen to seventeen. During my time, there wasn't a class that taught us about dealing with disappointment. However, leading to the age of fourteen and fifteen when decisions were being made in regards to receiving scholarships, they spoke to us about different options available if you do not get a scholarship. They informed us about other football clubs who would be willing to take you on if you are released. They also inform you about the option of going abroad or going to lower leagues. As a coaching staff, they reassured us that we were good enough and that we would make a living in the sport.

I received a scholarship at the age of sixteen. I completed my first year at West Ham but I was released by the club. I went to Barnsley FC to complete the remainder of my two year scholarship.

## How did it feel when you got released? How did you manage to deal with the mental challenges that came with the disappointment?

To be truthful, mentally, it took a big toll of me. I remember sitting with two other players and the manager. He told us that the Club was not willing to give us professional contracts half way through the two year scholarship. I was absolutely gutted because I believed that I had another year to prove myself. I thought they made their decision too early. I recall leaving the training ground that day and my dad picked me up. He consoled me and reminded me that it was not over. It was not the end! Personally, I thought my career in football was over. I questioned whether I was good enough to continue playing, especially at the elite level I was aspiring to play at.

I was fortunate to have the support of family and friends. This is what gave me the strength to pick myself up to go to Barnsley to finish my scholar there. I was grateful to them and their encouragement because going there provided the opportunity to continue playing professional football at an elite level instead of hanging up my boots.

## What advice would you give young aspiring footballers who may not play an elite professional level?

First and foremost, I would encourage them to have the self-confidence to pursue their dreams. In life, without self-confidence, you cannot be the best you can be. Sometimes as a footballer, you have to possess a certain arrogance. You have to believe that regardless of the competition, I know that I am good enough to get to where I want to be.

Secondly, I would inspire the message of hard work. I know of hardworking footballers who may not have been the most talented but because of their dogmatic work ethic went on to cement a good career in the sport. These two traits are important keys to becoming a professional footballer.

Confidence is something that anyone can develop. I personally do not believe we are born with confidence. I can't imagine a baby being born an intuitively knowing that he/she is 'ready'. You need good people around you. However, if you do not have that, you must demand that from yourself. I constantly remind myself to give the best I can. Evidently, if I fall short, I will not have any regrets because I gave everything I had and then some. Self- confidence is something that can be built up.

## How do you remain resilient in the challenging field of football?

For me, my faith plays a big role. I am a Christian. My life is for Christ, I am bold and happy enough to say that. Without faith I do not know how I would be able to continue. In football you can have good and bad days. You must have a thick skin. If you do not have thick skin, you will not last long in the game. To possess resilience is something that could take you from having two or three years in the game to eight or nine years. Every day **you must strengthen yourself physically and mentally. I must tell yourself 'no matter what happens, I will keep fighting to the end.'**

## How do you relate faith and hope in terms of your journey as a footballer?

Faith and Hope go hand in hand. I believe **hope is the foundation for lots of athletes and sportsmen and women.**

Without the hope to be someone great, you do not have the aspiration to push harder. Especially with footballers and mental health, if you do not have a hope to believe in yourself, mentally, you will not be able to cultivate a strength. **This is the life I have chosen. I will continue to take hits. It will hard. Its not uncommon to see footballer have career ending injuries, but without hope you will not be able to come back from a certain injury.**

As sportspeople and people in general,
we need to have hope!

Having a hope as a footballer gives
you the chance to be successful and
to have a career.

Our hope in ourselves, has to be strong!

**Why do you think men do not like to discuss the topic of health especially mental health?**

Us men seem to have an ego and a problem of pride when it comes to taking care of our health. We must put this aside to thick about the bigger picture -our families. There are somethings that we are afraid of and dread will happen to us. **We need to be honest with ourselves and families. We have to put that ego and so called 'Manliness' aside.** We need to face our problems head on even if it is life threatening. It's a case being prideful.

We must learn to lay down our stubborn
attitudes as men and humbling
ourselves to be honest and open.

We need to be honest with ourselves and families. We have to put that ego and so called 'Manliness' aside. We must be accountable to

**Following the death of your father from Cancer
twenty months ago, how have you dealt / are
you dealing with the mental challenges?**

My dad passed away as a result of having Prostate Cancer. His passing was a very traumatic time. I remember the day like it was yesterday. I felt nothing but anger. I do not remember being more angry in my life. I recall seeing him in hospital, I got so angry. I did not know what to do. I grabbed a chair and bent the bars of it. It was like a bad dream that I wanted to end.

In terms of coping with it, my family and I have coped with it well. It is not by our strength but only by God. Myself, my brother and mum have not had any counselling. We have not had any one to one counselling with specialist following the bereavement. Our council has been God, The Bible and the Holy Spirit. The pain had numbed as the days have passed. We were reminded of many good things that my dad did whilst he was alive.

Mentally, I'm ok.

I do not think I will ever get over it. I will always have memories of the experience. IN terms of my present demeanour, I am at a point where I can look forward to the future. My dad was a strong and fierce person but he was also very humble. The unique mix is something that resonates with me.

My dad was my coach, my manager,
the one person that always
believed in me.

Sometimes, coaches would tell me not to do certain things. However, my dad would advise me otherwise.

He is the reason why I still play football. I remember the day he passed, I told my brother that I am done with football. I will never step on the pitch again. In my mind, I could not do it without my dad. He was at every match I played. I realise now that to hang my boots would be the biggest regret because of the work my dad put in for me to get me here.

Moving forward, my hope and inner strength comes from the innate knowledge that I am doing this not just for God but also for my Dad. I have no choice but to make it as an elite footballer. I am not going to stop until I make a good living in the game.

One advise my dad gave me is *you have to do exceedingly more than anyone else. In doing so will get what you deserve.'* My dad was a big advocate of hard work and not being lazy. He used to say

*'Always think about the end result.'*

This is particularly meaningful when I reflect during days where things do not seem to go my way.

# Cancer

Cancer is a condition where cells in a specific part of the body grow and reproduce uncontrollably. The cancerous cells can invade and destroy surrounding healthy tissue, including organs.

Cancer sometimes begins in one part of the body before spreading to other areas. This process is known as metastasis.

More than one in three people will develop some form of cancer during their lifetime. In the UK, the four most common types of cancer are:

- breast cancer
- lung cancer
- prostate cancer
- bowel cancer

There are more than 200 different types of cancer, and each is diagnosed and treated in a particular way. You can find links on this page to information about other types of cancer.

## Spotting signs of cancer

Changes to your body's normal processes or unusual, unexplained symptoms can sometimes be an early sign of cancer.

**Symptoms that need to be checked by a doctor include:**

- A lump that suddenly appears on your body
- Unexplained bleeding.
- Changes to your bowel habits

But in many cases your symptoms won't be related to cancer and will be caused by other, non-cancerous health conditions.

**Reducing your risk of cancer**

Making some simple changes to your lifestyle can significantly reduce your risk of developing cancer.

For example:

- Healthy eating
- Taking regular exercise
- Not smoking

# Cancer treatment

Surgery is the first treatment to try for most types of cancer, as solid tumours can usually be surgically removed.

Two other commonly used treatment methods are:
chemotherapy – powerful cancer-killing medication
radiotherapy – the controlled use of high-energy X-rays.

# Conversation with Professor of Men's Health

**Professor Alan White**, PhD, MSc, BSc(hons), RN

Emeritus professor of Men's Health; Founder and Co-director of the Centre for Men's Health at Leeds Beckett University.

www.alanwhitemenshealth.co.uk

## What's your association with mental health? Have you directly experienced or know anyone/have encountered anyone with a mental health issue?

I have not worked within a mental health setting. After I graduated as a nurse in 1982 most of my clinical experience was in Intensive Care and other acute hospital settings. However, when I was Chair of the Men's Health Forum we did a lot of work on promoting men's mental health, with a number of high profile national campaigns. In 2010 I co-edited the only text focused onto the mental health of men: Conrad & White (2010) Promoting men's mental health (https://www.amazon.co.uk/Promoting-Mental-Health-David-Conrad/dp/1846193311).

I have a couple of other papers published (attached) and I was an Advisory Group member of the Victoria Medical Centre (Atlas) Men's Well-being Clinic, which was aimed at men in crisis. Our research centre also undertook for Movember a review of the current research evidence and practical ('tacit') knowledge about the core elements that make for successful work with boys and men around mental health promotion, early intervention and stigma reduction.

(https://cdn.movember.com/uploads/files/2015/Misc/
Promoting_MentalHealth_%26_Wellbeing_FINAL%5B2%5D.pdf)

In 2016, I had a 4 month period off work as a result of exhaustion and
acute anxiety due to overwork. During that time, I was able to benefit
from a rest and counselling and the coming to realise that my workload
was unsustainable. Thankfully I was able to get back to work and it was
not necessary to have medication.

## What inspired you to establish and co-direct 'Centre for Men's Health'?

As a nurse I have always been very aware of gender as an issue, especially
as a staff nurse on a female surgery ward. However, when I became a
lecturer on a nursing degree and then it's course leader it came to me how
little was done on men and their health in the curriculum. It inspired
me to look at how men managed to deal with a major health event
(experiencing chest pain) and what links could be made to masculinity
and male socialisation relating to their health and wellbeing. I soon
realised that there was very little research done on men and their health
(mid 1990's) and it prompted me to join the Kirklees Men's Health
Network (which was pioneering in its time) and from there the Men's
Health Forum (www.menshealthforum.org.uk), which was still part of
the Royal College of Nursing.

As the Forum developed it moved away from the RCN and became an
independent charity, with me as the Chair of the Board of Trustees,
I am now proud to be it's Patron. My research also progressed, with
amongst other studies undertaking the Scoping Study on Men's Health
for the then Public Health Minister in 2001. As our research developed
I applied to the University for a Personal Chair in Men's Health, which
was awarded and from that we developed the Centre for Men's Health.

Through the Centre we were able to help shape the way the discipline of
'men's health' was shaped globally. Unfortunately, the Centre was closed

by the University in the Summer of 2017 due to financial pressures and I am now semi-retired and continuing my work outside of the University. I was awarded Emeritus Professor of Men's Health status by the University, which retains my academic link, but I am now working mostly freelance. This includes being a member of the core group at WHO (Europe) as they prepare their first Men's Health Report and Strategy, which will be launched in the Autumn of 2018.

## What was the reason behind leading an international team of academics to conduct research regarding 'The State of Men's Health in Europe Report'?

We had been lobbying the European Commission for a number of years over the issue of men's health and they responded by putting out a tender for this report. I pulled together an international team and was successful in our bid. This was an exceptional opportunity to make a statement about men's health across the 34 countries we covered. This was the first official document from the European Commission on men's health and it created a lot of interest when it was published. There are two versions of the report, the first being the shorter official European Commission version, the second being the extended version, which has much more detail included.

(https://ec.europa.eu/health/sites/health/files/population_groups/docs/men_health_report_en.pdf; https://ec.europa.eu/health//sites/health/files/population_groups/docs/men_health_extended_en.pdf)

## What factor does having a mental illness have in relation to an individual attempting suicide?

It is recognised that there are people who are more at risk of suicide, such as those with depression, substance-abuse, personality disorders, schizophrenia and anxiety disorders.

Ex-military men that are suffering from post-traumatic stress disorder and the difficulty of re-acclimatising to civilian life are also at risk.

However, not everyone who attempts suicide would class themselves as having a 'mental illness'. There are certain occupations that see more suicides, with men working in the construction industry having nearly 4 times higher risk than the national average, with skilled tradesmen having double the national average of suicides. In these occupations there is greater job insecurity, with low pay, and lower socio-economic status, with the potential for multiple stressful life events. The recent recession has seen a big increase in the number of suicides in men. Men who have been abused as a child and have lost their partner, either through divorce or widowhood are also at greater risk.

There are also higher numbers of suicides in men who are gay, bisexual and transsexual, which may be linked to depression, but is also linked to issues of acceptance, belonging, stigma, and also bullying and victimisation.

## What are sportsmen's attitude to maintain and dealing with their mental wellbeing?

Can sports help to maintain a good mental health? (this is in relation to your work with the Premier League Health Initiative and Leeds Rhinos. Sport is a key part of many men's lives, both as a player and as a supporter and can have a significant role in their mental health.

Elite sportsmen and women can show great mental resilience, but when faced with emotional difficulties can be at greater risk of mental health problems, such as addiction, and suicide. It is important to work with all athletes on their emotional coping as at any time they could find themselves out of the game. There are now also sad cases of where even elite sportsmen and women have been the victims of abuse by coaching and medical staff.

Sport can provide an excellent opportunity to reach out to supporters to provide support and help to those with physical and mental health difficulties, with some excellent initiatives. One of the earlier examples was Premier League Health, which used the 'power of the club badge' to get young men engaged in a health programme that was run within the majority of the English Premier League clubs. The Football Fans in Training (FFIT) run within the Scottish Premier League was another example. A great mental health initiative was run within football – 'It's a Goal', with a current pilot going on within Rugby League by State of Mind Sport.

## Why do you think suicide rates amongst men are higher than women?

Although the number of suicides is higher in men it is important to note that suicide is also the biggest cause of death in women under the age of 34 years. Both men and women come to an ultimate feeling that they have lost everything and they have no other alternative, why there are so many more men that feel this way may be a result of women having greater awareness of the support systems in place to offer help and a stronger social network where they can discuss their problems.

Evidence from studies with boys from early childhood onwards show that they are under social pressure not to share when they are facing mental and emotional issues; this can persist into adulthood leaving men unprepared and disabled when having to deal with difficult emotional pain or anguish. This can also mean they are unable to recognise when help could be beneficial, resulting in them being isolated and alone in their struggle against the challenges they are facing. For many men a suicide attempt is not a cry for help, but a means of ending their life, so more leathal methods are used, such as hanging.

## Are men more susceptible to mental illness than women?

Men have higher levels of severe mental disorder, such as Schizophrenia, paranoia, psychotic disorders, which have a strong basis for diagnosis based on very problematic behaviour and symptoms. Women tend to have higher levels of bipolar affective disorders, anxiety and depression. Men have higher numbers of bed days than women for mental health disorders and be more likely to be sectioned under the mental health act.

There is a social class factor that needs to be considered when looking at the prevalence rates of depression and anxiety, where as many men as women who are living in the poorest communities are diagnosed.

It has been estimated that half of all lifetime cases start by 14 years of age and 75% before the age of 24 years[1]. It is also important to note that boys are more at risk of nearly all the developmental disorders, such as Delayed reading, Stammer, Attention deficit hyperactivity disorder, Tourette's Syndrome, Autistic spectrum disorders, Hyperkinetic disorders, Asperger's syndrome and Disruptive behaviour disorder, which can make them more at risk of mental health problems as they hit adulthood, if not directly, then through the impact of missed educational opportunities.

There is a possibility that many more men are showing signs of depression and anxiety but may be exhibiting their problems in different ways to those that are picked up by the usual diagnostic tools. In a study that used a more male sensitive set of questions there was an equal number of men as women diagnosed.

There are also men who have great struggles with their mental health that are missed. It is estimated that between 5 and 10% of new fathers suffer from post-natal depression.

---

[1] (Kessler RC, Berglund P, Demler O, *et al.* Lifetime Prevalence and Age-of-Onset Distributions of. *Arch Gen Psychiatry* 2005;**62**:593–602. doi:10.1001/archpsyc.62.6.59.

## Why is there a stigma regarding mental health? Where does this arise from?

There are two main forms of stigma, public stigma (relating to shared stereotypes relating to mental ill health) and self-stigma (where you personally believe in these stereotypes and act negatively as a result). They are mostly driven by fear of the unknown or from stories that are shared within communities about the possible causes and consequences of mental ill-health.

## Can the stigma be eradicated in its entirety?

It is hard to get rid of stigma as it can be passed on through so many different channels, with social media opening up new ways of reinforcing negative stereotypes and breeding hatred. Until we find ways of curbing these dangerous mediums stigma will persist.

## What are some of the ways we can address and change the stigma?

Schools are doing a great job of opening boys and girls eyes to the issues of mental health and the need to be understanding of their own and others emotional health be to be more accepting of different sexualities, ethnicities and religions. They are also introducing far more effective means of supporting boys and girls who are experiencing difficulties, such as through the use of counselling services. This not only gives immediate help, but also opens the eyes of those vulnerable to the opportunities for help as they grow older. The increasing media attention on the issue of mental health is so important as it helps normalise mental health and shows that you are not alone in your suffering.

It is also the responsibility of legislation to prevent discrimination of whatever form and wherever it is found, as we need to allay those fears of what will happen if a male or female has a mental or emotional health issue.

## What does hope mean to you? How can hope be associated with mental health?

**Hope is a very powerful construct that is closely linked to a belief that life is, or can be, good and that whatever difficulties you might be facing at this time there are better times ahead.** It is very hard keeping a sense of proportion when life seems full of difficulties and instilling a sense of hope into others who may have lost sight of that more positive future is a key aspect of friendship and therapy.

## How do you personally maintain a positive mental health?

I enjoy my work, and now I am out of the University and more in control of my own destiny and I can hopefully create a more manageable work-life balance. I still have some way to go ...

Not being too hard on myself (self-compassion), allows me to have bad days without feeling as if I have somehow failed. It also gives me permission to share any problems with my family and to discuss difficulties with my GP if necessary.

## What advice would you give to someone experiencing mental ill health?

Share with others your difficulties and be open to using professional support. Men who have engaged with talking therapies have found great success and if medication is needed it is to be welcomed and not avoided. There is no disgrace in being unwell, and we should accept care for our mental and emotional help in the same way as if we were diagnosed with diabetes, or a heart problem.

There is excellent male sensitive support now available, including the resources available from the Men's Health Forum, The CalmZone (CALM), and Movember. The Samaritans and Mind have to be seen as two of the most important free and immediately accessible services in the support of those most at risk. It is also really beneficial having social networks where you can be with others and to share a common sense of achievement or difficulty, rather than having to face it on your own. There are some amazing community initiatives aimed at men, that are not 'health' focused, but have great impact on emotional and mental wellbeing. Men's Shed's, gardening, organised walks all allow men to be with others and to talk in informal settings. There are also some great mental health initiatives being run through sport – the State of Mind work that is being done with Rugby League (http://www.stateofmindsport.org) being an excellent example.

Resources:

Men's Health Forum: Beat Stress, Feel Better https://www.menshealthforum.org.uk/beat-stress-feel-better
CALM- https://www.thecalmzone.net
Mind - https://www.mind.org.uk
Samaritans - https://www.samaritans.org/
Movember - https://uk.movember.com/about/mental-health
State of Mind Sport - http://www.stateofmindsport.org
Andys Man Club - http://andysmanclub.co.uk
Men's Sheds UK - https://menssheds.org.uk
Gardening groups - https://www.rhs.org.uk/communities/Find-a-group-search-form
Walking groups - http://www.ramblers.org.uk/go-walking/group-finder.aspx

Hope is a very powerful construct that is closely linked to a belief that life is, or can be, good and that whatever difficulties you might be facing at this time there are better times ahead

# Post-traumatic stress disorder (PTSD)

Post-traumatic stress disorder (PTSD) is an anxiety disorder caused by very stressful, frightening or distressing events.

Someone with PTSD often relives the traumatic event through nightmares and flashbacks, and may experience feelings of isolation, irritability and guilt.

They may also have problems sleeping, such as insomnia, and find concentrating difficult.

These symptoms are often severe and persistent enough to have a significant impact on the person's day-to-day life.

## Symptoms of PTSD

The symptoms of post-traumatic stress disorder (PTSD) can have a significant impact on your day-to-day life.

In most cases, the symptoms develop during the first month after a traumatic event. However, in a minority of cases, there may be a delay of months or even years before symptoms start to appear.

Some people with PTSD experience long periods when their symptoms are less noticeable, followed by periods where they get worse. Other people have constant, severe symptoms.

The specific symptoms of PTSD can vary widely between individuals, but generally fall into the categories described below.

## Re-experiencing

Re-experiencing is the most typical symptom of PTSD. This is when a person involuntarily and vividly re-lives the traumatic event in the form of:

- flashbacks
- nightmares
- repetitive and distressing images or sensations
- physical sensations – such as pain, sweating, nausea or trembling

Some people have constant negative thoughts about their experience, repeatedly asking themselves questions that prevent them from coming to terms with the event.

For example, they may wonder why the event happened to them and if they could have done anything to stop it, which can lead to feelings of guilt or shame.

## Avoidance and emotional numbing

Trying to avoid being reminded of the traumatic event is another key symptom of PTSD. This usually means avoiding certain people or places that remind you of the trauma, or avoiding talking to anyone about your experience.

Many people with PTSD try to push memories of the event out of their mind, often distracting themselves with work or hobbies.

Some people attempt to deal with their feelings by trying not to feel anything at all. This is known as emotional numbing. This can lead to the person becoming isolated and withdrawn, and they may also give up pursuing activities they used to enjoy.

## Hyperarousal (feeling 'on edge')

Someone with PTSD may be very anxious and find it difficult to relax. They may be constantly aware of threats and easily startled. This state of mind is known as hyperarousal.

Hyperarousal often leads to:

- irritability
- angry outbursts
- sleeping problems (insomnia)
- difficulty concentrating

# Conversation with a Territorial Army Reserve

**Justice Addison,**
*Web developer, Territorial Army Reserve*

## Who are you? What do you do for a living?

I work as a Web Developer by trade. I am also an active member of the Army Reserve (formally the Territorial Army). About five years ago, I joined as an infantry man, which is essentially the Army's 'man on foot with a rifle on the front line', also known as foot soldiers.

## Why did you join the Reserves?

I've always like the idea of being a soldier through films and literature. I like the idea of defence, i.e. defending one's country and people. This is something that attracted me to the role. I was also interested in building myself in discipline and physical endurance, so I was motivated by the fact that my physical capabilities would be challenged.

## What has been the positives and drawbacks?

I enjoy working with other people to achieve a common aim. I enjoy the teamwork element of the role. In my five years of service, I have been to four countries. Cyprus, Spain, Estonia and America to train, which means I encounter different cultures and work with different people. It has also helped to build leadership skills although I am not in a leadership position myself, I have been exposed to methods of leadership.

For me, the main drawback is the culture. There is a general culture where language use involves much swearing and sexual undertones to conversations. Many conversations are often filled with filth. Because of my belief and faith, I cannot always participate in certain conversations and the negative social activities because I do not fit. For me, this has been the main challenge of being in the army. I find these environments where such conversation take place not to be wholesome.

## Has being in the army has an effect in terms of how you manage your mental wellbeing?

The excitement I get from doing exercises provides mental stimulation which I think is positive. However there are moments where you get very tired and very little sleep and no signs of things stopping, which can be demoralising.

However, at the same time, you're usually with a group of people who are experiencing the same thing, therefore, a sense of comradery and companionship does help a lot. Where a mutual trust and friendship can develop as a result of spending days and nights together.

Even in spite of what I said about certain negative cultures, there is something about spending a lot of time with the same group of people to achieve a common goal which can be rewarding. Although I may not have much in common with some of the guys, having a common goal to fulfil ultimately brings us closer together. For me, I find this very fulfilling.

In terms of the negatives, again the influence of the culture can sometimes leave me in a place where I am unsure what to do or how to react. Part of the culture includes as element of 'banter' which involves a playful yet sometimes unwholesome teasing remarks amongst the infantry. There's a saying that goes something like 'you becoming more like the those you hang around'. I am conscious of this and there is a temptation of joining in the unsavoury conversations and activities at times for the sake of trying to fit in. At the same time, I know who I am. There is a constant battle in regard to what I can get involved with.

**If you were to look at society, the people in the military are perceived as 'hardcore' 'men's men'. Is there any room to express feelings of stress and anxiety? Would that be seen as a weakness?**

Generally, there is an undertone of not showing weakness. Being vulnerable is not what you want to express as such, you would be very careful who you disclosed certain information to. I have witnessed people become very stress and flipped out of control but some people turn it into banter and tease each other about it; laugh about it; perhaps as a coping mechanism.

When it comes to deeper issues, I do not think it is an environment where one can easily open up about things.

They do try to promote the concept taking to the chain of command if anything is bothering you. However, whether or not people use it, I wouldn't know.

Additionally, there is also the Padre, who is usually a priests or chaplain, who is available for people to talk to. Although the term originally had Christian roots, it is generally used today in military organisations to describe all professionals specially trained to serve any spiritual need, regardless of religious affiliation. They do not only attend to religious matters, but all aspects of wellbeing.

Therefore, there are some structures in place to help with mental wellbeing, but personally, I have not seen it being used much. In saying this, I would not know if the structures had been utilised as this would be done in confidentiality.

## Why do you think is it harder for men to speak about vulnerabilities?

In my view, there is an element of pride and not wanting to look weak. To add to this, there is also an element of not wanting to be judged. Everyman wants to appear as though they have it all together and can fight their own battles, which can be inhibiting – I find this is the case with me sometimes.

## How do you personally manage and maintain a positive mental wellbeing?

For me, it helps that I'm in the Reserves, which means I spend relatively little time away from my wife that I would have in the regular army. At any point I find it comforting to know that I'll soon be returning to my wife to talk to her. I also have a great Church network and a good group of friends I regularly hang out and play games with, which helps a lot. I also find achieving tasks and goals at work (or even generally) keeps me happy and in a positive mental state.

## Having read things about life after military service, I have sometimes come across Post Traumatic Stress Disorders (PTSD) – this is a mental illness which can often involves anxiety and depression. Why is / has PTSD become higher amongst people post army service? What tools are there to help such people?

I haven't yet been deployed to fight in war so it would be difficult for me to comment on this with a level of experience. I have heard others speak about it who have been in that situation. When you are involved in war, because of the nature of it, you find little time to process what is going on. The is a lot that happens in battle that can be overwhelming, i.e. seeing casualties of war; perhaps even terrible treatment of civilians;

seeing your friends injured or killed; hatred; violence; etc, yet a soldier has to be entirely focused on the task at hand.

I think these unprocessed events can build up and compound with time. It is only afterwards when you are removed from the environment that these things come back in full force, which leaves the individual not knowing how to deal with it.

When you are in a situation of war, you are there to perform a duty of service and that duty has to be paramount otherwise you could put the mission at risk of failing.

War is not good.

## What does hope mean to you? How do you relate hope to what you do in the army?

Many people have hope in the national army. If the nation came under some measure of attack, I believe civilians would place their hope in the military to help and defend them. In as much as sometimes I feel the British public are not keen on the Army and its expense, people do still have hope in it.

For me, having the skills to be able to stand up if anything happened gives me a certain amount of confidence.

In America, people in the military are treated very differently. When I was training there, people would frequently approach us on the streets, thanking us for our service. I found the attitude to be quite different there than in the UK.

I cannot however separate hope from my belief in God. Ultimately my hope is to be with Christ and to experience his fullness one day and the joy and peace that come with that. There is a portion in the Bible which states that "He will wipe every tear from their eyes. There will be no more death' or mourning or crying or pain...". My hope is in God, and whenever I am going through a saturation, I try to have this I mind. When I do, it spurs me on to try and overcome the difficulty.

**For me this is the ultimate hope.**

Many people have hope in
the national army.

I think the army does bring
hope especially in the currently
climate of political unrest.

# CONVERSATION WITH BUSINESS SYSTEMS, DATA AND PRODUCTION MANAGER

**Nana Amofa,**

BSc (Hons) CAIA

I have been indirectly encountered mental health issues. My first encounter with mental health was when a close relative of mine (person A) began to exhibit changes in their typical behaviour pattern. The strange thing about this was, these weren't your far left, easily identifiable, stereotypical outbursts that unfortunately have come to be associated with mental health, but rather slight divergences from what I and the family were used to. In our case, it was excitement and caution. Things that were moderately humorous were extremely hilarious to them and things that were seemingly normal to the vast majority triggered an overly cautious and suspicious response.

At first we dismissed it, rather chalking it up to a fleeting blip, an outlier that would soon fade however, this was not the case. As a month went by, their behaviour became more erratic, such that we were witnessing memory loss, a strange desire to not be in the dark, urges to reorganise their home coupled with the caution and suspicion mentioned previously. Swiftly moving through the account, I was now accompanying the family member to appointments with a specialist doctor. At first, the doctor was unable to diagnose them due to that fact that during the doctor's sessions none of the aforementioned symptoms were displayed. We would attend the sessions and person A would be a completely different person, they would be the person that they wanted the doctor to see. After many repeat visits, and accounts from others, the doctor decided to prescribe aripiprazole, which began the path to recovery. Albeit a short account, the process from initial symptoms to recovery would take 6 months, but

I strongly believe this would have taken much longer had we not detected it when we did.

## Men

I cannot say for certain why men may find it difficult to talk about mental health, but I would assume that it may come down to the stereotypical dominant and in control image placed on men. Due to this image, when a man is now faced with mental health, it would mean admitting that you are not in control, and this can be a frightening experience, especially when you are not fully informed of the changes you are undertaking.

The social stigma associated with mental health is unfortunately often one of weakness, and this can be challenging for a man, as this would mean confessing a weakness and accepting that we are not altogether rounded as we like to think.

## Hope

Hope is the confidence to look forward, unbound by the limitations of today. For me, hope meant there would be a day when we would look back at this and we would have crossed the bridge. Hope allowed me not to be overcome with dismay when the situation dictated the contrary.

## Stigma

Education can help to eradicate the stigma. People typically fear that which they do not know. The more we educate ourselves and others around us concerning mental health, the more we can accommodate and foster and new approach towards mental health.

Being a Christian, my positive outlook on life is predicated on the Bible and the Good News it brings to all mankind. I believe that with Christ I am never defeated and because of Him I can win at life every day.

# CONVERSATION WITH A PSYCHIATRIST

Dr TBS Balamurali,

*Consultant Psychiatrist in East London*

**What is your experience regarding Mental Health i.e.**
**What does your role / duties involve as a psychiatrist?**

Currently I manage a male inpatient 19-bedded open ward.

Most of those admitted there suffer from serious mental disorders – schizophrenia, bipolar disorder, extreme personality disorders, but also depression, suicidality, anxiety disorders and PTSD. Often these are complicated by alcohol or illicit substance abuse. With the increased focus on community care and cut to overall budgets, those admitted now tend to be at the more serious end of the spectrum.

Patients are admitted usually via A&E, GP referrals, or through contact with the police or Criminal Justice System, with some coming in from Mental Health Act Assessments arranged in the community We assess them and treat them with medication, talking therapies, other therapies as indicated, and advise and support them to manage financial, social and other stressors they may experience in the community.

However inpatient services are only a small part of the overall care provided to those with mental disorders. As services are currently set up – there are also community mental health teams who provide longer term care to those with severe mental disorders, in the community. There is also a team who work with GPs in their surgeries to see and advise on those presenting with milder mental health disorders, who may not necessarily need longer term complex input.

Additionally there are other specialised mental health teams – notably the crisis team, who provide short-term intensive support at home to those with acute mental health problems, as an alternative to hospital admission.

Apart from this there are numerous other statutory and voluntary services out there to help those in distress, or who need support with alcohol or other substances, or social factors, and an extensive provision of talking therapies as part of the IAPT – Improving Access to Psychological Therapies.

## Comment of how mental health issues is portrayed in the Media / Arts (film / theatre). Does this accurately represent how it is in real life?

I feel, and I'm sure most of my colleagues agree, that there is a major problem in the way mental health issues are portrayed in the media and arts.

The vast majority of those with mental disorders are not dangerous to others, and you are actually far more likely to be harmed by someone you know, without a mental health problem. The media chooses to sensationalise mental disorder, as this makes better reading, and similarly cinema and theatre has been guilty of this, without adequate research into the true nature of mental illness. We understand the artistic need to make a story interesting, but feel that there is a responsibility for an artist or journalist to accurately represent mental disorders and their treatment.

Those with mental illness are already subject to huge stigma and misportrayal can only add to this, leading to those with mental illness feeling marginalised and misunderstood, and less likely to be willing to accept their illness or seek treatment, thus compounding the problem. Fortunately there have been huge leaps forward, and the BBC and many theatre companies have made specific efforts to address this issue, but we have a long way to go.

## Causes and symptoms of mental health? What are the available treatments? – Medication / Psychotherapy etc.

Mental disorders have a multifactorial cause. Most professionals would agree with the stress-vulnerability hypothesis, such that each one of us has various vulnerabilities within us, due to genetics or upbringing / environment, which combined with a particular stressor, is likely to cause a disorder. This does not only apply to mental disorder. For example, you are far more likely to break a leg if you have weak bones for whatever cause (the 'vulnerability') and/or extreme pressure is applied to the bone (the 'stress'), than without either. (In fact you will not break your bone without one or both in combination – bones do not break for no reason).

Mental disorders can manifest in a huge variety of ways – too many to comprehensively list here. However the main features to note would be a sustained disturbance of mood, such as being elated or low in mood, disturbance of your functioning, such as your memory, or ability to care for yourself or fulfil social duties, paranoia, a change in your social interactions and behaviour, or most obviously hearing or experiencing things that did not happen (hallucinations) or believing things that are not true without adequate reason for your belief (delusions).

Treatment is multifactorial. Most psychiatrists use the bio-psycho-social model. Using this we will seek to address any biological factors, treating any physical health issues and prescribing medication as indicated; psychological treatments such as CBT or psychotherapy may be indicated if the individual has certain disorders and is amenable to engage with a talking therapy; and social factors such as problems with housing and finance and safety etc.

## Trend of mental health illnesses over the last 25 - 50 years. Why have the rates of diagnosis increased?

It is difficult to know if the increase in diagnosis is due to an actual increase in the prevalence of mental illness, or that levels of mental illness are the same, but we are better at diagnosing and treating them.

We would hope that with improved healthcare and less inequality, the actual incidence would be lessening, but things associated with mental disorder such as alcohol use and illicit substance abuse are increasing, as well as the possible breakdown in society that has been much bemoaned. It may be that incidence is actually increasing because life appears to be more stressful, despite overall improved quality of life according to most measures.

What does seem to be the case is that rates of detection of mental disorders are increasing. This must be due to greater awareness amongst the public and professionals, and discussion amongst the media and celebrities regarding their own mental health. Additionally the government has increasingly recognised the importance of mental health and there has been much discussion in parliament about the importance of mental health.

## Views on stigma and mental health. Is this stigma worse in some cultures / ethnicities (Afro-Caribbean / Asian)?

Studies to seem to indicate that there may be higher rates of mental disorder among certain ethnic minorities, and that the stigma associated with identifying and treating mental illness are certainly worse in many, more traditional societies.

We do not know whether mental illnesses rates are higher in some groups due to the stress of migration, or that those with a tendency to mental illness may be more likely to migrate, or that they may have had more stressful experiences in their homeland leading them to migrate, or that the stress of being 'other' to the surrounding society after migration increases likelihood of developing mental illness. The increased rates seem to persist into second-generation immigrants.

Once ill however, there seems to be much resistance to accessing services, perhaps due to different formulations of mental disorder, as being spiritual disturbances, rather than medical conditions. Even if considered medical disorders, the acknowledging of this may lead to stigma and ostracisation of the individual and possibly the family.

Additionally attitudes mean that certain groups appear particularly unlikely to utilise available services such as talking therapies. Much work is being done to educate and inform people about what treatments are available and how to access them, but this still relies on people recognising that there is a disorder there.

Hope is the confidence to look
forward, unbound by the
limitations of today

# What to do if we're experiencing mental health issues.

*"I would suggest that the first place to go to would be your GP to discuss what you are experiencing and ask for help. In an acute crisis, you can attend any emergency department in a hospital.*

*If you feel you need to talk to someone, chat to friends or family, or an organisation such as the Samaritans. Often people are scared of opening up about their feelings but usually feel better after doing so, and indeed talking to someone who understands, about what you are experiencing, is part of the treatment of mental disorders.*

*If you really feel unsafe you should contact the police.'*

# RESOURCES

Mental health charities, groups and services in the UK.

## Mental Health Foundation
**020 7803 1101**

Improving the lives of those with mental health problems or learning difficulties.

## Together
**020 7780 7300**

Supports people through mental health services.

## The Centre for Mental Health
**020 7827 8300**

Working to improve the quality of life for people with mental health problems.

## Depression Alliance
**0845 123 2320**

Provides information and support to those who are affected by depression via publications, supporter services and a network of self-help groups.

## British Association for Counselling and Psychotherapy
**01455 883300**

Through the BACP you can find out more about counselling services in your area.

## PANDAS Foundation
**0843 28 98 401 (every day from 9am-8pm)**

PANDAS Foundation vision is to support every individual with pre (antenatal), postnatal depression or postnatal psychosis in England, Wales and Scotland. We campaign to raise awareness and remove the stigma. We provide our PANDAS Help Line, Support Groups offer online advice to all and much more.

## General advice and support

### Citizens Advice
Gives free confidential information and advice to help people sort out their money, legal, consumer and other problems.
Support for children and young people

### Young Minds
**020 7336 8445**
Provides information and advice for anyone with concerns about the mental health of a child or young person.

### Childline
**0800 1111**
Free, national helpline for children and young people in trouble or danger.

### Nightline
Listening, support and information service run by students for students.
Other places you could go for support

### Age Concern
**0800 009966**
Infoline on issues relating to older people.

### Lesbian and Gay Switchboard
**020 7837 7324**
Provides information, support and referral services.

### Refugee Council
**020 7346 6700**
The UK's largest organisation working with refugees and asylum seekers.

## Relate
**0300 100 1234**

Offers advice, relationship counselling, sex therapy, workshops, mediation, consultations and support.

Counselling Directory A free, confidential directory of trained, professional counsellors and therapists in the UK

## Teacher Support Network
**08000 562 561**

A 24/7 telephone support line which gives teachers access to professional coaches and counsellors 365 days a year. The network also campaigns for change within schools and education policy in order to improve the wellbeing, mental and physical health of teachers.

## Anxiety UK
**08444 775 774**

Works to relieve and support those living with anxiety disorders by providing information, support and understanding via an extensive range of services, including 1:1 therapy.

## Mind
**0300 123 3393**

Provides advice and support to empower anyone experiencing a mental health problem. We campaign to improve services, raise awareness and promote understanding.

## Samaritans
**116 123 (UK)**
**116 123 (ROI)**

We're here round the clock, 24 hours a day, 365 days a year. If you need a response immediately, it's best to call us on the phone. This number is FREE to call. You don't have to be suicidal to call us. We'll talk about difficult issues We don't skirt around issues, and we're not afraid to go into deep and difficult areas. Sometimes just having the acceptance from someone that what they say won't be judged is enough to help people open up.

*Dear reader,*

*Thank you for taking your time to read this book. It is my sincere desire that you have learnt something useful. To those who are suffering from some sort of mental ailment or those of you who know someone that is a sufferer; though this illness is still very much misunderstood and stigmatised, please know that you are not alone! There is support out there if you are courageous enough to reach out. I beseech you not to lose hope!*

*Do not ever lose the audacity and the courage to keep hoping even through the most difficult of moments.*

*I wish you all a perfect mental health!*

# About The Author

*Emmanuel Owusu is the author of 'My Psychosis Story', 'Let's talk mental health' and 'The Arts and Mental Health'. Having been diagnosed with a life changing mental illness in his early twenties in 2015, he was sectioned under the Mental Health Act 1983. This culminated with him spending a month in a psychiatric hospital in London, England. Following his ongoing recovery, he sought to learn more about his diagnosis and mental health as a whole. His journey has led him to publish a series of books and articles in relation to mental health. Emmanuel has a passion for helping raise awareness of mental health issues in the hope that it educates people which will help reduce the stigma within society.*

# NOTES